THE
AUTOIMMUNE
KETO
COOKBOOK

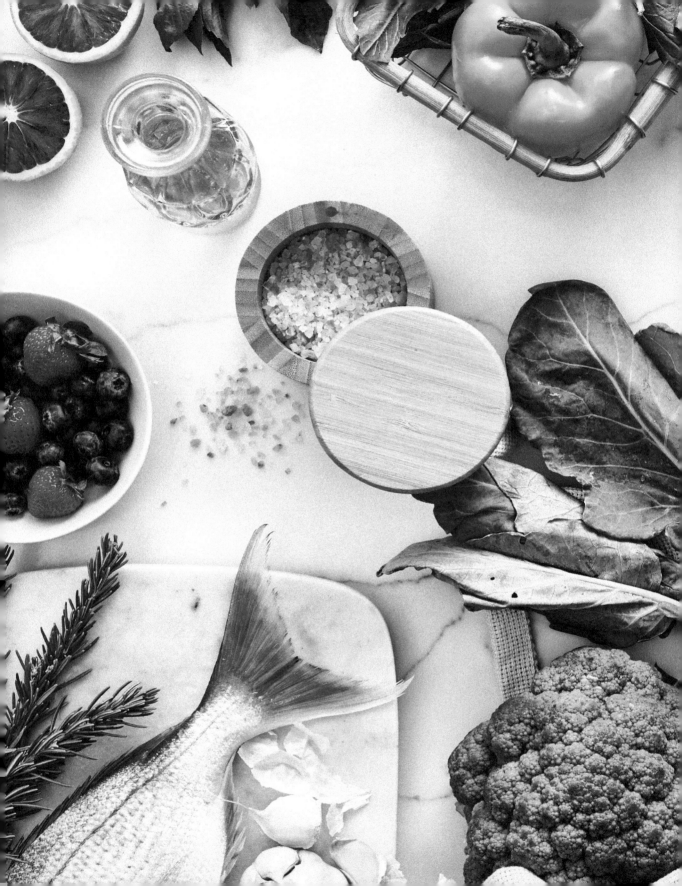

THE

AUTOIMMUNE
KETO
COOKBOOK

Heal Your Body with Delicious AIP-Compliant
Recipes and Meal Plans

KARISSA LONG & KATIE AUSTIN

Photography by Alicia Cho

ROCKRIDGE
PRESS

For general information on our other products and services or to obtain technical support, please contact our Customer Care Department within the United States at (866) 744-2665, or outside the United States at (510) 253-0500.

Rockridge Press publishes its books in a variety of electronic and print formats. Some content that appears in print may not be available in electronic books, and vice versa.

TRADEMARKS: Rockridge Press and the Rockridge Press logo are trademarks or registered trademarks of Callisto Media Inc. and/or its affiliates, in the United States and other countries, and may not be used without written permission. All other trademarks are the property of their respective owners. Rockridge Press is not associated with any product or vendor mentioned in this book.

Interior and Cover Designer: Richard Tapp

Art Producer: Karen Williams

Editor: Claire Yee

Production Editor: Jenna Dutton

Photography: © 2019 Alicia Cho

Food styling by Ashley Nevarez

Cover image: Cucumber and Beef Mint Salad p104

Author photo courtesy of © Alexandra Strimbu

ISBN: Print 978-1-64611-038-4 | eBook 978-1-64611-039-1

R0

TO OUR FAMILIES

FOR BEING THE ULTIMATE SUPPORT SYSTEM

THROUGHOUT OUR HEALING JOURNEY.

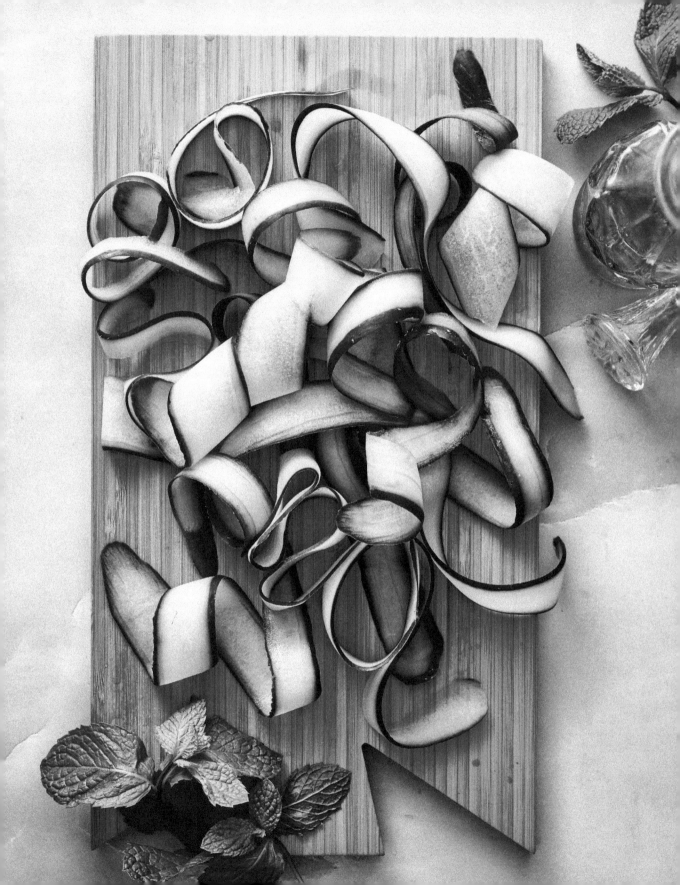

CONTENTS

INTRODUCTION

Welcome to *The Autoimmune Keto Cookbook*! We are so thrilled that you have picked up this book to learn how the power of nutrition and ketosis can help heal your body. If you are reading this introduction, you most likely have been diagnosed with an autoimmune disease or know someone who has. While an autoimmune diagnosis can be extremely scary, frustrating, and even debilitating, we have good news for you! There is hope, there is a path to healing, and there is a way to live well with an autoimmune disease. How do we know this? Because we are *living proof*!

Between the two of us, we have four autoimmune diseases, including ulcerative colitis, Hashimoto's thyroiditis, postural orthostatic tachycardia syndrome, and ankylosing spondylitis with symptoms including fatigue, joint pain, heart palpitations, bleeding, cramping, and digestive distress. We lived with these symptoms for years while our doctors continued to write us prescriptions for medicines designed to treat our symptoms but not heal the root cause.

It wasn't until we went on our own quest for answers that we truly began to understand the importance of food as it relates to our health. We spent years poring over medical research, studying nutrition science, and experimenting with different dietary theories until we finally found a way to eat and live that not only put our respective autoimmune diseases into remission, but also healed our bodies and enabled us to achieve optimal wellness.

Our health journeys were a winding road of wins and setbacks, trials and errors. But ultimately, these experiences allowed us to create and refine a blueprint for others suffering from autoimmune diseases to easily follow in order to achieve life-changing results. Our passion to share this blueprint with as many people as possible led us to launch Clean Keto Lifestyle, a company focused on helping others live their best lives by utilizing the power of ketosis.

When it comes to our diagnoses and our subsequent wellness journeys, we have very similar stories and we are quite confident that many others do as well. That is why we wrote this book. So that someone one who has just been diagnosed with an autoimmune disease or someone who has been suffering with one for years, or anyone in between, can learn the exact process that we have used in our own lives to achieve incredible outcomes.

In the following chapters, we'll provide you with a comprehensive plan for healing your body inside out! In Part One of this book, we'll explain the background and science behind Autoimmune Keto, what steps you should take to prepare, and provide three weeks of meal plans to get you started. In Part Two, we share 85 delicious recipes that are designed to nourish your body while at the same time getting it into ketosis.

By the end of this book, you will have all the tools and resources you need to start living an Autoimmune Keto life. We can't wait for you to get started and truly begin to take your health into your own hands.

xo,
Karissa & Katie

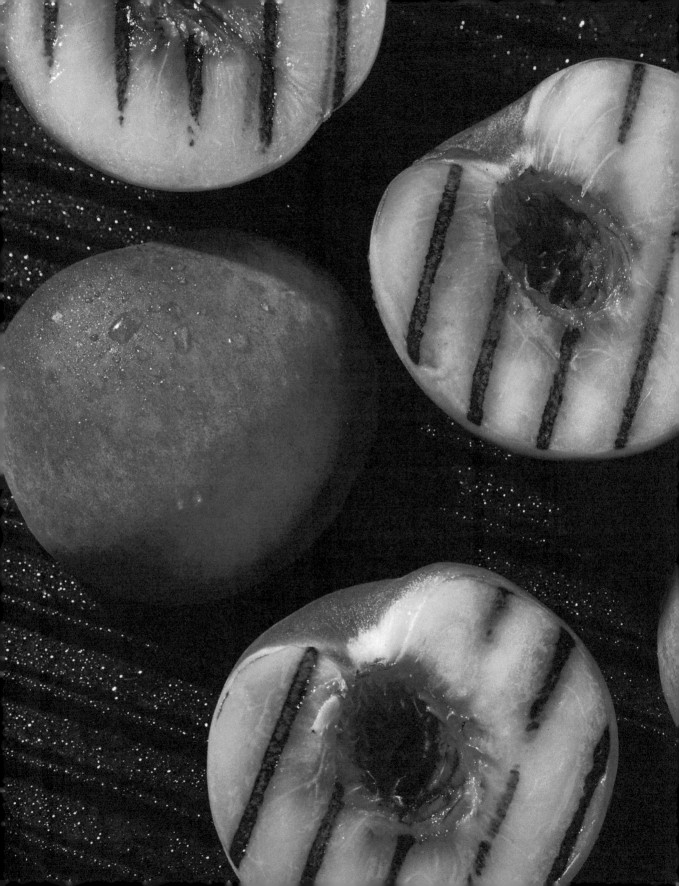

PART ONE

TREATING AUTOIMMUNE DISEASES THROUGH KETO

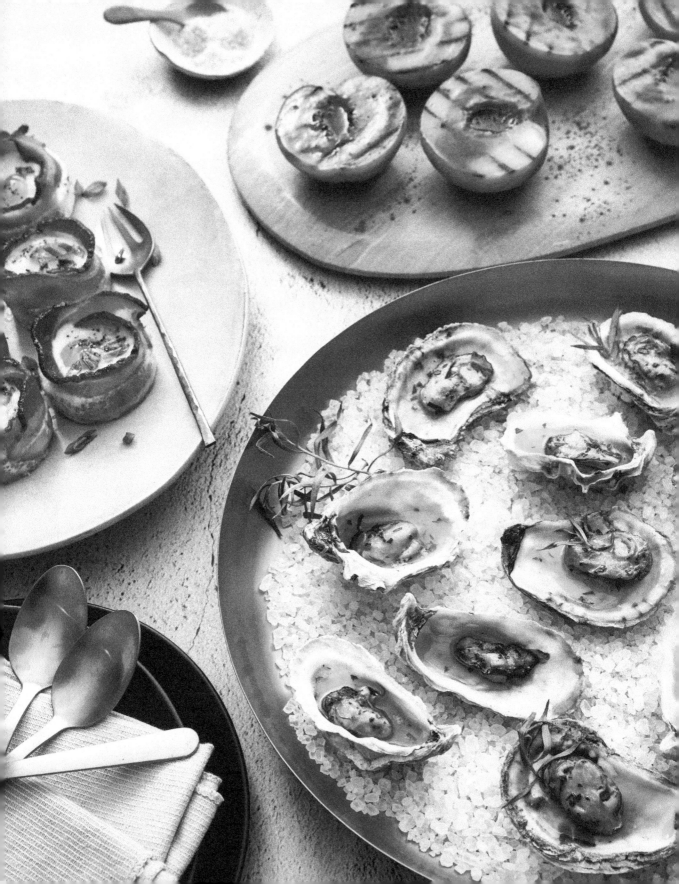

Chapter 1

THE LINK BETWEEN
AUTOIMMUNE DISEASES AND DIET

Your diet is an integral part of your health. This is especially true when you are suffering from an autoimmune disease. This chapter explains the link between autoimmune disease and diet so that you understand how powerful food can be when it comes to your well-being. We believe that information is power, especially when you're about to embark on a wellness journey!

What We Know About Autoimmune Diseases

More likely than not, you know someone who has been diagnosed with an autoimmune disease. According to the American Autoimmune Related Diseases Association (AARDA), more than 50 million Americans suffer from autoimmune diseases, and this number grows on a daily basis.

The AARDA defines an autoimmune disease as a varied group of illnesses that affect almost every human organ system, including our nervous, gastrointestinal, and endocrine systems, as well as our eyes, skin, blood, and blood vessels. In all of the more than 100 autoimmune diseases identified, the underlying problem is "autoimmunity," meaning the body's immune system becomes misdirected and attacks the organs it was designed to protect.

Here are some of the most common autoimmune diseases:

- Addison's Disease
- Celiac Disease
- Chronic Lyme Disease
- Endometriosis
- Fibromyalgia
- Graves' Disease
- Hashimoto's Thyroiditis
- Inflammatory Bowel Disease (IBD), which includes Crohn's Disease and Ulcerative Colitis
- Lupus
- Multiple Sclerosis
- Psoriasis
- Rheumatoid Arthritis
- Scleroderma
- Type 1 Diabetes
- Vitiligo

The range of symptoms varies by disease and individual—and can come and go, making autoimmune diseases sometimes tough to diagnose—but the most common ones are fatigue, swelling, achy muscles, joint pain, and brain fog.

Autoimmune diseases are a relatively new form of disease, with the first diagnoses occurring around the 1950s, so the medical community is just beginning to understand all the factors involved. Research has identified several common causes that contribute to autoimmunity:

Genetics – Genetics play a huge role in all aspects of your health, which is particularly true in immunity function. It is quite common for multiple members of a family to have an autoimmune disease since they share a similar genetic makeup. If you're already diagnosed with one autoimmune disease, you are more susceptible to develop additional autoimmune diseases as your genes are more predisposed to autoimmunity.

Diet – Your diet plays a significant role when it comes to developing an autoimmune disease. What you eat and drink (both the types of foods and the quality) can create conditions within your body that increase your risk for an autoimmune disease. These conditions include leaky gut (also known as permeability in your intestinal wall), increased and chronic inflammation, vitamin and nutrient deficiencies, and an overstimulated immune system.

Lifestyle – Factors such as chronic stress, poor sleep, and lack of movement all have the ability to increase your risk for autoimmune disease. Each of these factors or a combination of them can impact your body's immune function and contribute to developing autoimmune diseases.

Environment – Your body is constantly being exposed to chemicals, bacteria, pathogens, viruses, and other toxins within our environment. These toxins lurk in our homes in the form of cleaning products, skincare items, and makeup, to name a few. They lurk in our food in terms of pesticides, herbicides, antibiotics, and GMOs. They can even exist in our water supply in the form of chlorine, lead, and even arsenic. This regular exposure can trigger the development of autoimmune diseases.

When it comes to treating autoimmune disease, all of these contributing factors should be considered.

How the Immune System Works

Simply put, the immune system is designed to protect your body from harmful threats such as pathogens, toxins, parasites, bacteria, viruses, and other microbes.

It is an intricate system made up of multiple organs and thousands of cells that work collectively to fight off invaders and remove them from the body.

There are two primary parts of the immune system, which work together as your body's protector:

Innate Immune System – This is the immune system that you are born with. It is the first responder when your body identifies an invader. It rapidly goes into action and surrounds the invader to kill it.

Adaptive Immune System – This is the immune system that you develop throughout your life, as your body is consistently exposed to pathogens, toxins, parasites, bacteria, viruses, and other microbes. After your body is invaded, the adaptive immune system produces antibodies designed for each specific invader after the first exposure. These antibodies remain in your body in order to defend against that same invader next time it enters the body.

What Goes Wrong with an Autoimmune Disease

As long as your body's defense system is working properly, your immune system will go unnoticed. Problems begin to occur when your immune system creates antibodies that end up attacking your own healthy cells and organs, not just the invaders. Essentially, your own body's immune system can't tell the difference between healthy cells and invaded cells, so it becomes misdirected and attacks what it was designed to protect, which leads to various autoimmune diseases depending on what organ or group of cells it targets. For instance, rheumatoid arthritis is the result of your immune system attacking your joints, ulcerative colitis develops from inflammation in your colon, and psoriasis is a function of your skin cells being under attack.

How Diet Affects Your Autoimmune Disease

Your diet can be a significant contributing factor—for better and for worse—to the development of an autoimmune disease. Emerging research now links gut health with our immune system function. Since your gut health has a direct correlation to what you are feeding your body, it is imperative to focus on your diet when attempting to manage your autoimmune disease.

There are various aspects that need to be addressed when it comes to your diet and autoimmune disease:

Inflammation – Inflammation is always present in our bodies. Some is advantageous—for instance, your body uses inflammation to heal when you get a scrape or a bruise. However, chronic inflammation can become a problem, especially when it comes to immune system function. Much of the foods available to us in a modern diet contain additives, artificial ingredients, preservatives, and sugars that promote inflammation within the body. This consistent stream of inflammation-producing foods puts a strain on our bodies and overstimulates our body's immune system.

Vitamin & Nutrient Deficiency – Most of us know that vitamins and nutrients are essential to your health, but what you may not know is that they also have a significant influence on your immune system. Unfortunately, as people continue to eat processed foods over whole foods, it's common to lack essential nutrients, minerals, and vitamins. This lack of nutrients strains our immune systems, which can lead to autoimmunity.

Microbiome – The human microbiome is made up of trillions of living microorganisms, including bacteria, yeast, fungi, and viruses. The health of your microbiome, especially as it relates to your digestive tract or gut, is pivotal when it comes to regulating your immune system function. An imbalance in your microbiome can make your body more susceptible to autoimmune disease.

Food Allergies & Sensitivities – To paraphrase an old saying: One person's medicine can be another person's poison. This is especially true when it comes to food. Each person reacts differently to the foods they consume and subsequently digest. If you are eating foods that your body is allergic, intolerant, or sensitive to, you could be triggering your immune system.

In order to properly treat and manage your autoimmune disease, it is crucial that you address your diet. The great news is that you can *absolutely* do something about what you're eating. With just a few changes and upgrades to your food choices, you will be well on your way to healing!

How Keto Works

Now that you understand the link between diet and autoimmune disease, let's talk about the ketogenic diet, a large part of the foundation that will start you on your path to healing.

The ketogenic diet is a low-carb, moderate-protein, high-fat diet designed to exhaust glucose levels and prompt the body to provide an alternative source of energy to the brain. These alternative energy sources are called ketones, which are produced by the liver using stored fat. The keto diet has mainly been touted for its weight-loss merits, but is often overlooked for how powerful and effective the diet is for improving your overall health. The key is to implement the keto diet the right way. Let's review the basics:

Ketosis

Ketosis happens when the body takes stored fat through the liver and produces ketones (small molecules used as fuel throughout the body). When your body is in a state of ketosis, it literally becomes a fat-burning machine.

INFLAMMATION AND LEAKY GUT

"Leaky gut" has become a common phrase in the medical community as it plays a significant role in inflammation and autoimmunity. Leaky gut occurs when the lining of your small intestine weakens, allowing contents to cross the intestinal wall and enter your bloodstream or lymphatic system. These contents can include toxins, bacteria, viruses, or other undigested particles. Once your immune system recognizes these foreign items, it immediately goes into action. This constant activation of your immune system causes inflammation in your body, which creates an immune response that can lead to autoimmunity.

The good news is that a leaky gut can be treated and repaired. That's right, you can reseal your intestinal lining through diet and lifestyle improvements. Many people find that by just addressing their leaky gut, some or all of their autoimmune symptoms subside.

Macros

How do you get into ketosis? It all comes down to what you eat and how much you eat of each specific macronutrient (also known as "macros"). There are three types of macronutrients in the human diet: fats, proteins, and carbohydrates. On the ketogenic diet, your daily macronutrient breakdown should be as follows:

- 75 percent fat
- 20 percent protein
- 5 percent carbohydrates

That's right—approximately 75 percent of what you eat each day will come from fat. Fat is the most essential macronutrient that the body needs. You need fat to live and it is 100-percent necessary for you to get into ketosis.

Food Quality

Aside from the macronutrient ratio guidelines, an important (and often disregarded) part of keto is *food quality* and centering your diet around food that encourages healing. We like to break down these foods into three categories:

Healthy Fats

There are many different varieties of fat ranging from healthy to downright dangerous for you (e.g., trans-fat and hydrogenated oils). Because the ketogenic diet is centered around fats, it is vital that you are consuming the right ones! The fats you ingest should be from whole, unrefined foods such as olives, avocados, and coconuts. Healthy fats should come from the farm—not factories—and have no added ingredients. When available, always opt for organic versions to limit your exposure to GMOs, pesticides, herbicides, and other toxins.

Quality Protein

Eating quality protein is critical for everyone, regardless of what diet you are on. Conventional protein sources today (meat, poultry, eggs, and seafood) that are the most widely available to consumers are also most likely mass-produced, factory-farmed, and unhealthy for you. Most of these animals (even the fish!) are raised in conditions that are overcrowded and dirty. To control disease, these animals are pumped full of antibiotics. They are also fed a grain-based diet, which results in inflammation, depleted nutrients, and high instances of omega-6 fatty acids (the bad kind if too high) in the animals. Remember, at the end of the day, "You are what your food eats!" so it is vital to understand where your protein is coming from and how it is raised.

Our definition of quality protein means sourcing and consuming grass-fed beef, pastured poultry and eggs, heritage-breed pork, and wild-caught seafood. It is 100-percent worth the extra effort to find and purchase quality protein. It is necessary for your health to eat the most nutrient-dense, clean protein available.

Organic Veggies

Organic vegetables will make up the majority of all the carbs you consume on the ketogenic diet. You need to eat vegetables on keto to ensure you are getting sufficient fiber, vitamins, and minerals. When picking your vegetables, opt for the non-starchy variety and make sure they are organic whenever possible.

Organic produce is grown and processed without bioengineered genes (GMOs), synthetic pesticides, petroleum-based fertilizers, and sewage sludge–based fertilizers. Organic vegetables have higher antioxidant, vitamin, and mineral content than their conventionally grown counterparts. Oftentimes, when people with intolerances to chemicals or preservatives switch to eating only organic vegetables, they find that their symptoms lessen and even go away.

How Keto Helps Autoimmune Diseases

Implementing a ketogenic diet with a focus on the *quality* of the food you are consuming each day can help with autoimmune diseases because it addresses several of the root causes of autoimmunity.

Reduced Inflammation – A huge benefit of being in ketosis is that it can lower inflammation. Free radical production, which is extremely inflammatory, is reduced when burning ketones for energy. Additionally, when you remove processed foods from your diet like you do with our keto approach, you end up eliminating the consumption of all inflammation-producing additives, artificial ingredients, preservatives, and sugars. When you replace these processed foods with real foods, these nutrient-dense powerhouses work to decrease internal inflammation in your body.

Improved Gut Health – By implementing keto using our quality standards, you consequently stop consuming all forms of sugar, gluten, starches, and other grains that can be extremely irritating to your small intestine lining and contribute to leaky gut. By substituting these types of foods with foods that promote gut healing (healthy fats, bone broth, quality proteins, and fermented veggies), you can slowly repair your intestinal lining.

Increased Vitamin & Mineral Consumption – Fat plays a crucial role in vitamin and mineral absorption. It needs to be present when ingesting fat-soluble vitamins (vitamins A, D, E, and K) so that they are properly absorbed by the body. Since your diet is 75-percent fat when eating keto, your body's ability to absorb vitamins and other nutrients significantly increases. When you couple this improved absorption with all the nutrient-dense vegetables and proteins that you consume on keto, you'll find that you have an effective formula for restoring your body's essential vitamins and nutrients and re-regulating your immune function.

Other Benefits

Achieving and maintaining ketosis by implementing the keto diet with quality foods is the best way for humans to operate most efficiently. Being in ketosis can lead to additional benefits such as weight loss, more energy, improved focus, better sleep, clear skin, strength gain, reduced appetite, better digestion, and balanced mood. Many of these benefits also have a positive impact on immune system function.

What Is Autoimmune Keto?

Now that we have the basics of the ketogenic diet down, let's take it to the next level with our version of **Autoimmune Keto**. Autoimmune Keto combines the principles of the ketogenic diet with the elimination and reintroduction methods of the Autoimmune Protocol (AIP).

Whereas the goal of the ketogenic diet is to get your body into ketosis, the goal of AIP is to eliminate and reintroduce food categories over a period of time in order to identify food allergies, intolerances, or any other sensitivities that could trigger autoimmune disease symptoms. Similar to keto, the foods that you eat while implementing AIP are whole foods designed to restore your body's nutrients and promote healing.

The combination of keto and AIP can be extremely powerful in treating autoimmune disease symptoms, reducing inflammation, and ultimately healing your body. Autoimmune Keto creates the foundation for you to begin your wellness and recovery journey. This method worked for both of us to overcome our debilitating autoimmune diseases. As a result, we are extremely passionate about the merging of these two dietary theories that complement each other incredibly well.

Understanding the Autoimmune Protocol (AIP)

So, what exactly is AIP? In simple terms, AIP calls for the elimination, for a period of time, of all food categories that are commonly found to be problematic for people with an autoimmune disease. These foods include the following:

- Grains and Starches
- Beans and Legumes
- Dairy
- Eggs
- Nuts
- Seeds
- Nightshades
- Alcohol

During this *Elimination Phase*, all of these foods are removed from your diet, along with any artificial ingredients, sweeteners, or processed foods. You will also add in various foods that promote gut health and are extremely nutrient-dense. These foods include:

- Bone broth
- Gelatin or collagen from grass-fed sources
- Wild-caught seafood
- Fermented foods

After you have seen significant improvements in your symptoms and reestablish a good health baseline, you can then slowly reintroduce foods back into your diet. During this *Reintroduction Phase*, you will begin to consume the foods that you initially eliminated one-by-one and assess how your body reacts. This phase is very informative and should be performed systematically so that you can learn what foods your body can tolerate. At the end of this phase, you will have crafted a customized and long-term solution for your diet. The entire process is very empowering as you listen to your body, understand its health cues, and build a deeper connection to your inner intuition.

Why Choose Autoimmune Keto?

During our personal wellness journeys to heal our autoimmune diseases, we both started with AIP on its own. While implementing AIP, we found our symptoms gradually improving, but something was missing from our healing process. We were constantly hungry and experienced energy ups and downs throughout the day. Following this intuition, we began to evaluate what we were eating on a daily basis and quickly identified that on AIP, we were still consuming large amounts of sugars (albeit natural sugars in the form of fruits, honey, and maple syrup) and we weren't eating enough *fat*!

AIP didn't provide any sort of macronutrient guidelines and instead only included guidelines on what you could eat and what should be avoided. Once we started researching suggested macros, the ketogenic diet came into the picture.

Our initial reaction to the keto diet was that there was significant overlap of the types of foods you could eat between keto and AIP. All we really needed to do was up our fat intake (a lot!) and lower the amount of natural sugars we were consuming. These changes were straightforward, and we found that adding keto into our lifestyle was relatively seamless. As soon as our bodies got into ketosis, we noticed our healing sped up! At the same time, implementing AIP became so much easier because all the healthy fats we were eating on keto kept us full and satisfied and reduced our cravings. It was a win-win!

One of the most common questions we get is "Do you need to do both methods in order to see results?" We wish there was a black-and-white answer to this question, but truthfully the answer is that *it depends on the person*. For some people, keto alone works well to manage their autoimmune disease symptoms, while others may need both AIP and keto. It really comes down to your individual health needs.

We think Autoimmune Keto is the most efficient method because it provides a baseline for you to then measure your progress. It also removes all immune-provoking foods—so you won't be keeping anything in your diet that could potentially make your symptoms worse.

If you think implementing AIP and Keto together will be too restrictive, we recommend starting with keto. Once you achieve ketosis, which usually takes between seven to ten days, and are reaping the benefits of reduced cravings and a controlled appetite, you can slowly move into the Elimination Phase of AIP. The Elimination Phase will be much easier to do if you aren't battling sugar and carb cravings, but rather just removing dairy, eggs, nut/seeds, nightshades, and certain spices from your diet. It is also important to note that if you start with keto and all of your symptoms subside and you feel great, there is no need to implement AIP.

Other Important Elements of Autoimmune Keto

We've said it already, but it is worth mentioning again: *food quality* is a necessity when implementing Autoimmune Keto. If you continue to feed your body nutrient-void processed foods, inflammatory-provoking refined oils, and foods full of toxins (pesticides, antibiotics, etc.), you will never fully heal your body.

Micronutrients and Vitamins

If you are suffering from an autoimmune disease, you most likely have some sort of micronutrient deficiency, which can include deficiencies related to fat-soluble vitamins, B vitamins, vitamin C, minerals such as iron, magnesium, and zinc, amino acids, and antioxidants. As a result, it is crucial that you eat a wide variety of foods that are rich in nutrients and provide the vitamins and minerals that your body needs to function optimally.

Choosing Nutrient-Dense Foods

In order to eat quality, nutrient-dense foods, you first need to source them. Lucky for all of us, finding foods that are farm-fresh, organic, and high-quality is getting easier and more affordable.

Here are our go-to tips for choosing nutrient-dense foods:

1. Look for the following quality indicators on the food label:

   - Fats: organic, unrefined, non-GMO
   - Proteins: organic, grass-fed, grass-finished, heritage-breed, pastured, wild-caught
   - Vegetables: organic, non-GMO, and local

2. Head to your local farmers' market: You can't beat the taste and nutrient profile of food that comes straight from a nearby farm. The shorter transport time ensures you are getting the food at its peak freshness. Make sure to seek out farmers who use organic farming techniques.

3. Shop online: Shopping online is a great option for people who don't have the ability to find quality foods at their local grocery store or farmers' market. It's also a good option for busy people who don't have the time to go to the store each week and like the convenience of getting food shipped directly to their front door. Our favorite websites are:

   - Amazon
   - Thrive Market
   - ButcherBox
   - Sizzlefish
   - NOW Foods

Making Autoimmune Keto Work for Your Body

Making Autoimmune Keto work for your body really comes down to three simple things:

Commitment – In order for you to achieve amazing results with Autoimmune Keto, you have to actually *implement* it. That means you need to commit to the process and follow the food and macronutrient guidelines detailed in this book. Don't put too much pressure on perfection or let it paralyze you, but do make a pledge to yourself that you will do everything in your power to stay on this healing path.

Patience – Everyone's body has different needs, especially when it comes to the range of autoimmune diseases that exist. Be patient! You didn't get sick overnight, and your body won't heal overnight. Keep in mind that each day on Autoimmune Keto is one more day of you making progress.

Honesty – Be honest with yourself. Trust your instincts and the cues your body is giving you. This is especially true in the AIP Reintroduction Phase. As you go through the process of adding back foods one at a time, be truthful about what is working and what is not. The goal is to create a personalized plan that *works* for your body. During this phase, we suggest that you use our *Reintroduction Phase Worksheet* on page 49 to track and figure out which foods work or don't work for you.

How to Use This Book

This book is designed to set you up for success when it comes to Autoimmune Keto. We have each been through our own personal healing journeys with autoimmune diseases and have taken everything that we've learned and incorporated it into this book. We're going to give you all the tools that you need to heal your body from the inside out, minimize/eliminate your autoimmune symptoms, and truly live well!

First, we are going to start with preparation, which is essential for success. In the next chapter, we will guide you through choosing the right foods, planning your macros, prepping your meals, and stocking your kitchen.

Once you are prepped and organized, we are providing you with three weeks of Autoimmune Keto meal plans designed to get you into ketosis while following the Elimination Phase of AIP. These meal plans were developed with nourishment and healing in mind, and come with shopping lists as well as weekend prep instructions to save you time.

Lastly, we are sharing more than 85 recipes that are both simple and delicious so that you always know what to eat and never feel stuck while doing Autoimmune Keto. All the recipes in this book are keto with the majority of them being AIP-Elimination Phase Compliant. We have also added several recipes that you can use during your Reintroduction Phase of AIP and have labeled them accordingly. To further help you with your personalized needs, we have added ingredient swap tips so you can customize the recipes to the phase that you are in.

By the end of this book, you will feel confident, prepared, and most importantly, motivated to start the Autoimmune Keto approach. This method completely changed our lives and transformed our health for the better, and we know it can do the same for you!

BEYOND DIET

Food plays an integral role in autoimmunity and healing, but there are also certain lifestyle factors that should be addressed in order to improve your health and minimize your symptoms:

STRESS MANAGEMENT

We have all experienced some form of stress, which is your body's reaction to change or a challenge. Chronic and consistent stress can lead to health problems such as internal inflammation, hormone imbalance, and even a weakened immune system. Managing your stress is very important with Autoimmune Keto. Here are some techniques that you can use:

- Practice meditation
- Get a massage or take a relaxing bath
- Pick up a relaxing hobby (painting, knitting, or gardening)
- Perform breathing techniques

MEANINGFUL SLEEP

Sufficient sleep is a MUST with Autoimmune Keto. Sleep is 100-percent necessary for your physical and mental health. Aim for at least seven to nine hours of sleep each night. Here are some tips for improving your sleep:

- Create a bedtime ritual and follow it each night, with the goal of going to sleep at the same time every night.
- Put down your phone and turn off the TV at least two hours before your bedtime to avoid blue light exposure that can be disruptive to your sleep cycle.
- Improve your sleep environment by making sure your bedroom is quiet, dark, and cool.

CONSISTENT MOVEMENT

Notice we didn't say *exercise* here. With Autoimmune Keto, we don't want you exercising too much and putting undue stress on your body. Over-exercising or consistently pushing your body too hard, too long, or too often can do more harm than good, so we just want you to focus on consistent movement such as:

- Go for regular walks outside with your family, friends, or your dog
- Practice yoga or try a Pilates class
- Play with your kids
- Stretch

It is important to note that you really need to listen to your body when it comes to physical activity. If you are feeling worn out or fatigued, slow down and rest.

EXPOSURE TO SUNLIGHT

For years now, we have been told to hide from the sun and slather on SPF at all times, but unfortunately the result of this advice is that more and more people are becoming vitamin D deficient. Vitamin D is essential for optimal heath and plays a large role in immune system function. Bottom line: you need vitamin D! The best and most natural way to get vitamin D is to expose your skin to sunlight. Here are our sun-safe tips:

- Limit your unprotected sun exposure to 20 to 30 minutes each day.
- Expose your skin to sunlight between 10:00 am to 2:00 pm when the sun is strongest and its rays are most intense.
- Expose as much skin as possible (arms, legs, stomach, face, chest).
- Aim for sun exposure at least three times a week.

For people who don't live near the equator, year-round sun exposure is not possible. In this case, vitamin D supplementation is necessary. We recommend getting your vitamin D levels tested and working with a doctor to determine the best supplement dosage for you.

CONTINUED

ELIMINATE TOXINS IN YOUR ENVIRONMENT

Toxins are not only in our foods, they're also prevalent in our household products, personal care items, and water supply. As we breathe these toxins, apply them to our skin, and/or ingest them, we activate our immune system. To truly heal our immune system function, we need to eliminate as many of these toxins as we can. Here is a list of the best ways to do this:

- *Swap out your cleaning supplies.* Have you ever noticed when you are cleaning your house with conventional cleaners that your eyes water, you have trouble breathing, or you start coughing or sneezing? These bodily reactions are a direct result of the chemicals lurking in your cleaning supplies. Opt for cleaning products that use essential oils, vinegar, and other plant-derived ingredients instead. Here are some of our favorite brands:

  ▸ The Honest Company
  ▸ Seventh Generation
  ▸ Branch Basics
  ▸ Mrs. Meyers

- *Upgrade your skin and makeup products.* Our skin is actually the body's largest organ and plays a crucial role in regulating our health. Every product that comes into contact with our skin has the potential of making its way inside our bloodstream. Unfortunately, most skincare, hair care, and makeup companies can and do use harmful ingredients in their products. These toxins include lead, parabens, phytates, and sodium laurel sulfate, which can disrupt your endocrine system and impair immune function. Do your body a favor and make the upgrade to clean beauty products. Here are our favorite places to shop clean beauty brands:

▸ Credo Beauty (www.credobeauty.com)
▸ The Detox Market (www.thedetoxmarket.com)
▸ Whole Foods Market (www.wholefoodsmarket.com)
▸ Honest Beauty (www.honestbeauty.com)

• *Filter your water*. Most standard tap water is not as pure as we think it is and can be contaminated with toxins such as chlorine, lead, and even arsenic. Since you can't control the quality of your municipal water, use water filters to protect yourself from potentially harmful contaminants. Depending on your budget, there is definitely a water filter option for you:

▸ Most affordable: water filter pitchers or faucet-attachment filters
▸ More expensive: whole-home water filtration systems

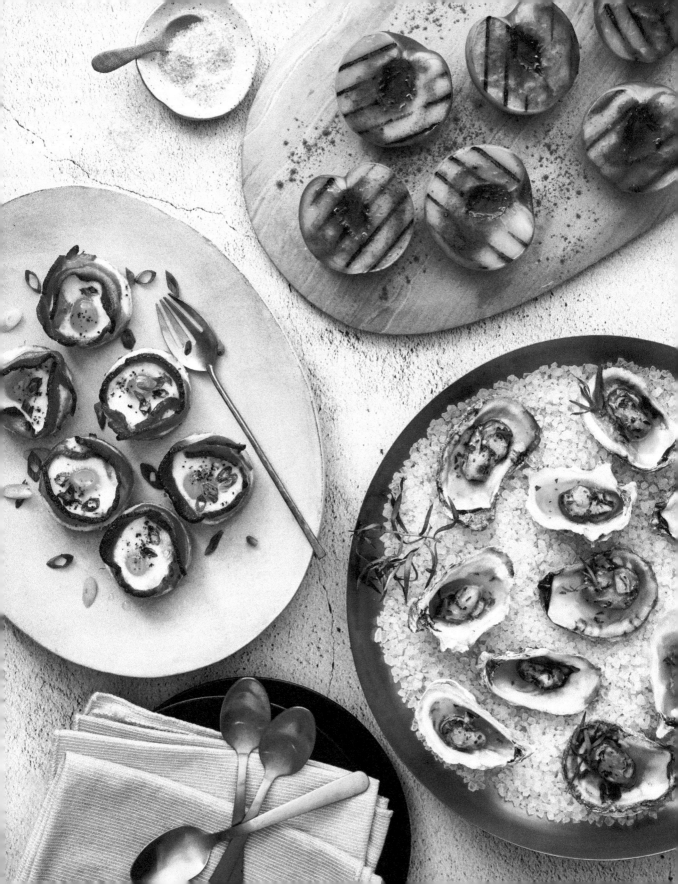

Chapter 2

SETTING YOURSELF UP
FOR SUCCESS

Now that we have gone through the science associated with Autoimmune Keto, it is time to get you set up for success! Like everything else in life, being prepared is the key. This chapter outlines the exact steps you need to take in order to start Autoimmune Keto. These steps include knowing what to eat and avoid, planning your macros correctly, prepping your meals, and stocking the right foods in your kitchen. This chapter also includes three weeks of meal plans so that you can easily follow them as you begin this new, healthy phase of your life!

What to Eat and Avoid

The goal of Autoimmune Keto is to eliminate and reintroduce food categories over a period of time in order to identify food allergies, intolerances, or any other sensitivities that could trigger autoimmune disease symptoms, while at the same time getting your body into ketosis. As a result, the table below incorporates *both* AIP and keto food guidelines into one comprehensive list. This will act as your reference guide throughout Autoimmune Keto. There are four sections in the table:

Foods to Eat Freely – These are foods that are both keto and AIP friendly, meaning you can and *should* eat these in abundance. Once again, remember quality is key! Opt for the highest quality and the most nutrient-dense foods available (see page 14 for the labels you should be looking for).

Foods to Eat in Moderation – These are foods that are AIP friendly, but have a higher carbohydrate and sugar content. Your daily intake should be limited to ensure it doesn't hinder your ability to achieve and maintain ketosis.

Foods to Avoid Initially but Can Be Reintroduced – These are foods that are removed from your diet as part of the Elimination Phase of AIP. As a result, these foods should be avoided initially, but can be added back during the Reintroduction Phase (see page 25 for all the details).

Foods to Avoid – These are foods that should be avoided because of their high carbohydrate content or because they promote inflammation.

Foods to Eat Freely

HEALTHY FATS

- Avocado
- Avocado oil
- Bacon fat (nitrate-free, no sugar added)
- Coconut butter, manna, or cream
- Coconut milk, full-fat
- Coconut oil
- Extra-virgin olive oil
- Lard
- MCT oil
- Olives

QUALITY PROTEIN

- Bacon (nitrate-free, no sugar added)
- Beef
- Beef gelatin powder
- Bison
- Chicken
- Collagen peptides
- Crab
- Duck
- Elk
- Halibut
- Lamb
- Liver
- Lobster
- Mussels
- Oysters
- Pork
- Salmon
- Sardines
- Scallops
- Sea bass
- Shrimp
- Squid
- Tripe
- Trout
- Tuna
- Turkey

NON-STARCHY VEGETABLES

- Artichokes
- Arugula
- Asparagus
- Bok choy
- Broccoli
- Brussels sprouts
- Cabbage
- Cauliflower
- Celery
- Chard
- Chives
- Cucumbers
- Endive
- Fennel
- Garlic
- Kale
- Leeks
- Lettuce
- Mushrooms
- Okra
- Onions
- Radicchio
- Radishes
- Rhubarb
- Shallots
- Spinach
- Sprouts
- Water chestnuts
- Zucchini

FERMENTED FOODS

- Kimchi
- Non-dairy kefir
- Sauerkraut

BEVERAGES

- Bone broth
- Filtered water
- Seltzer/sparkling water, unflavored
- Unsweetened herbal tea (black, green, chamomile, peppermint)

HERBS AND SPICES

- Basil
- Bay leaf
- Chives
- Cilantro
- Cinnamon
- Clove
- Curry
- Dill weed
- Garlic
- Ginger
- Horseradish
- Lemongrass
- Oregano
- Parsley
- Peppermint
- Rose
- Rosemary
- Saffron
- Sage
- Spearmint
- Tarragon
- Thyme
- Turmeric
- Vanilla (powder or gluten-free extract)

FLAVORINGS

- Capers
- Coconut aminos
- Fish sauce
- Pink Himalayan salt or Celtic sea salt
- Vinegars (apple cider, balsamic, red wine, and white wine)

Foods to Eat in Moderation

LOWER SUGAR FRUITS (MAX ½ CUP A DAY)

- Blackberries
- Blueberries
- Cantaloupe
- Cranberries
- Grapefruit
- Lemons
- Limes
- Peaches
- Pomegranate seeds
- Raspberries
- Strawberries
- Watermelon

NATURAL SWEETENERS (MAX 1 TSP EACH DAY)

- Coconut sugar (5 carbs per tsp)
- Molasses (5 carbs per tsp)
- Pure maple syrup (4 carbs per tsp)
- Raw honey (6 carbs per tsp)

Foods to Avoid Initially but Can Be Reintroduced

NIGHTSHADES

- Eggplants
- Peppers of all kinds (bell peppers, hot peppers, paprika, cayenne)
- Tomatillos
- Tomatoes

DAIRY

- Butter
- Buttermilk
- Cheese
- Full-fat yogurt
- Ghee
- Heavy cream
- Sour cream
- Whey

EGGS & EGG-BASED SAUCES

- Aioli
- Béarnaise
- Chicken eggs
- Duck eggs
- Mayonnaise

NUTS (INCLUDING NUT BUTTERS & MILKS)

- Almonds
- Brazil nuts
- Cashews
- Macadamia nuts
- Pecans
- Pine nuts
- Pistachios
- Walnuts

SEEDS (INCLUDING SEED BUTTERS & MILKS)

- Cacao
- Chia
- Cocoa
- Coffee
- Flax
- Hemp
- Poppy
- Pumpkin
- Sesame
- Sunflower

NON-AIP SPICES

- Allspice
- Anise
- Black or white pepper
- Caraway
- Cardamom
- Celery seed
- Coriander
- Cumin
- Dill seed
- Fennel seed
- Juniper
- Mustard seed
- Nutmeg

KETO SWEETENERS

- Erythritol (non-GMO)
- Monk fruit extract (100% pure)
- Stevia (100% pure)

LOW-SUGAR ALCOHOL

- Clear liquors
- Dry wines

Foods to Avoid

GRAINS & STARCHES

- Barley
- Buckwheat
- Corn
- Oats
- Quinoa
- Rice
- Rye
- Wheat

HIGHER SUGAR FRUITS (INCLUDING FRUIT JUICE)

- Apples
- Bananas
- Cherries
- Dates
- Figs
- Grapes
- Kiwis
- Mangos
- Oranges
- Pears
- Pineapple
- Plums

STARCHY VEGETABLES

- Butternut squash
- Plantains
- Potatoes
- Sweet potatoes

BEANS & LEGUMES

- Beans
- Lentils
- Peanuts
- Peas

HIGH-SUGAR ALCOHOL

- Beer
- Dark liquors
- Hard ciders
- Sweet wines

REFINED OILS

- Canola
- Corn
- Grapeseed
- Margarine
- Safflower
- Soybean
- Vegetable

REFINED SUGAR OF ALL KINDS

- Agave
- Brown sugar
- Evaporated cane juice
- High fructose corn syrup
- Powdered sugar
- White sugar

ARTIFICIAL SWEETENERS & DRINKS

- Energy drinks
- Equal
- Soda/diet soda
- Splenda
- Sweet 'n Low
- Truvía

Planning Your Macros

As part of Autoimmune Keto, you will be focusing on achieving ketosis. The secret to getting into ketosis is ensuring that you are eating the right combination of your macronutrient categories (75 percent Healthy Fats; 20 percent Quality Protein; and 5 percent Carbohydrates).

These percentages are daily goals, so each individual meal doesn't need to follow these guidelines exactly. We do recommend that you have fat at each meal to keep you satiated and provide for better vitamin and mineral absorption. And to be clear, the 5 percent carbohydrates should come from organic vegetables and low-sugar fruits—nothing from the *Foods to Avoid* list on page 26.

It is also important to mention that when it comes to carbs, we measure our macros using *net carbs*, which is calculated by taking total carbs less fiber. This is the measure of carbs that are actually absorbed by the body.

With Autoimmune Keto, we don't believe tedious macro tracking is necessary. Instead, we use a different technique called the 8-3-6 Formula, which focuses on serving sizes and how you are building your daily meals.

To follow the 8-3-6 method:

- Aim to eat 8 servings of fat each day – SERVING SIZE = 1 tablespoon
- Aim to eat 3 servings of protein a day for a total of 60 to 80 grams – SERVING SIZE = the size of your palm
- Aim to eat 6 servings of non-starchy vegetables – SERVING SIZE = 1 cup

THINGS WE WISH WE KNEW
BEFORE WE BEGAN

As you begin to embark on this Autoimmune Keto journey, we would like to impart some wisdom to you.

- **Enjoy Yourself.** Restoring your health doesn't need to feel like punishment or restriction. Switch your mindset and really embrace this journey. Remember, you are nourishing your body from all aspects.
- **Slow & Steady Wins the Race.** There is nothing wrong with starting slow, and we advise not trying to do too much too soon. If you are feeling overwhelmed, start in phases rather than doing everything all at once. This can mean starting with keto for a week or two and then moving into AIP or simply eliminating food categories one at a time.
- **Trust Your Instincts.** Listen to your body and follow your intuition. Through this process, you will build a deeper connection with your body.
- **Practice Self-Kindness.** Have compassion for yourself and don't beat yourself up if you have a setback, just start fresh the next meal or next day.
- **Pat Yourself on the Back.** Celebrate your successes and milestones and be proud of yourself every step along the way. Nothing is too small to celebrate!

Tracking macros really comes down to personal preference. Many people find this way of calculating their macros easier to maintain. Some people find meticulously counting macros works best for them. If you are in the latter group, you can figure out your personalized macros using an online calculator and then track your macros using a mobile phone app (MyFitnessPal is a good one). Each recipe in this book includes macro nutritional information for your convenience.

Prepping Your Meals

Meal prep is a critical step to success. By planning and prepping your meals ahead of time, you have a strategy. By the time you're ready for your meal, all the chopping, roasting, and other prep work will be done, and all that's left to do is assemble and eat!

Everyone's schedule is different, so figure out a time to prep meals that works for you. For the most part, you will need to carve out about one to two hours to get all your meal prepping done for the week. Most people opt to meal prep on Sunday, but if Wednesday night is when you have the most time, by all means, do it then. The key is making meal prep a part of your lifestyle and fitting it into your calendar. Like everything in life, the more you do it, the better you get, and the easier it becomes.

Make Easy Meals

The first trick to meal prepping is to not overcomplicate it. For the first few weeks, keep your meals simple. Pass on the complicated recipes, and instead opt for a smoothie at breakfast, a salad at lunch, and a roasted protein with veggies for dinner. The simpler your meals are, the easier and faster it will be to prep them.

Starting with simple meals that are easy to put together will give you good practice and build your confidence. Once you master the staples, you can add in new recipes that are more intricate.

Cook in Bulk

Cooking in bulk (aka batch cooking) is the most efficient way to utilize your time in the kitchen. When it comes to proteins, roast, bake, or poach your meats (chicken, beef, turkey, etc.) and seafoods (salmon, shrimp, tuna, etc.). Wash, peel, and chop your veggies, and then roast or steam them in a large batch. You'll also want to make sauces and dressings for use throughout the week.

Store your prepared food items in clear, sealed containers so you can locate them easily in the refrigerator. We recommend glass containers or BPA-free plastic. If you plan to bring meals to work with you, assemble them ahead of time. Pack up your roasted protein with some veggies, build a salad, and keep the dressing on the side; or blend up a smoothie and store it in the refrigerator.

Get Creative with Leftovers

When meal prepping, look for ways to utilize the same ingredients in your meals throughout the week or simply have the same meal more than once a week by cooking double or triple batches at a time. This way, you have fewer ingredients to buy and you can meal prep even more efficiently.

You can roast a whole pastured chicken at the beginning of the week for use in a delicious salad for lunch and then serve it with roasted vegetables for a satisfying dinner later in the week.

To some people, leftovers can be boring. Feel free to liven up your leftover meal up by adding some toppings like a drizzle of oil or fresh herbs. Another option is to serve your leftovers in a different manner, such as cold vs. warm or in a bowl vs. a plate. These little changes can trick your brain into thinking it is a new dish.

Stocking Your Kitchen

Having a well-stocked kitchen with these Autoimmune Keto staples will ensure you have the basics to whip up a quick meal at any time. Below are go-tos that you will always find in our kitchens.

REFRIGERATED ITEMS

- Grass-fed ground beef
- Pastured chicken thighs
- Salad greens (arugula, kale, or spinach)
- Vegetables (broccoli, cauliflower, zucchini)
- Wild-caught salmon

COUNTERTOP ITEMS

- Avocados
- Fresh herbs (basil, rosemary, cilantro)
- Garlic
- Ginger root
- Lemons/limes
- Onions

PANTRY ITEMS

- Apple cider vinegar
- Avocado oil
- Balsamic vinegar
- Coconut aminos
- Coconut milk, full-fat
- Coconut oil
- Extra-virgin olive oil
- Fish sauce
- Pink Himalayan salt

- Baking sheet
- Blender or food processor
- Cutting board
- Large pot
- Mixing bowls (various sizes)
- Parchment paper (look for the non-bleached kind)
- Saucepan
- Sharp knife
- Skillet
- Steamer basket

Your 3 Weeks of Meal Plans

We know from personal experience that any new way of eating works only if you enjoy the foods that you're consuming, the dishes are easy to make, and you feel *satisfied*. In other words, it has to be delicious and satiating but also practical. The following meal plans are designed to check off all three of these attributes!

These meal plans are meant for the initial Elimination Phase of Autoimmune Keto so that all the guesswork is removed and you know precisely what you can eat. You can follow these meal plans exactly, or you can use them and the recipes in Part Two of this book as a jumping-off point to plan your own meals.

Each weekly meal plan will include recipes, shopping lists, and weekend meal prep instructions to make sure you have all the tools you need to master Autoimmune Keto seamlessly. There are also ideas for snacks if you are hungry between meals. The key to Autoimmune Keto is providing your body an abundance of nourishing foods. Don't worry about counting calories and most importantly don't skimp on the *fats* in the recipes!

Meal Plan Notes

Servings Guidance

- To make it easy, the meal plans are designed for **one** person.
- Most recipes make one to three servings; check each specific recipe to be sure.
- For recipes that are more than one serving, cook the full recipe and save the additional servings for later meals throughout the week. We will note "leftover" meals on the plan.
- Adjust the recipe measurements accordingly if cooking for more people.

Food Storage

- Some recipes call for half a lemon or lime. Store the remaining half face-down on a small plate in the refrigerator to save for the next use.
- Put fresh herbs in a glass jar filled with about an inch of water. Cover with a plastic resealable bag and store in the refrigerator.
- Some recipes call for 1 cup of coconut milk (most cans have 2½ cups). If a recipe calls for less than 1 can of coconut milk, follow these steps:

  - Shake the can vigorously before opening to blend the solids and the water completely.
  - Open the can and measure out the amount needed.
  - Pour the remaining milk into a sealed container and store in the refrigerator for up to 5 days.
  - Bonus: Store 1 or 2 cans of coconut milk in the refrigerator at all times so you'll always have a cold can when you want to make a smoothie.

Making Substitutions

- If you don't like certain foods, feel free to swap them out of the recipes for an equivalent macronutrient on the Foods to Eat Freely list on page 23 (e.g., chicken for salmon or broccoli for asparagus).
- Make sure to adjust the cooking time and recipe instructions accordingly.

More Quick Tips

- Don't binge or stuff yourself. Eat until you are 80-percent full, not to the point of discomfort.
- If you work during the week, assemble or make your lunch the night before. Keep any dressing on the side—don't pour it over the dish until you're ready to serve it.
- A few of the recipes do include natural sweeteners such as honey, maple syrup, and coconut sugar. While these are not traditionally "keto," we have added them to some recipes for a touch of sweetness. The amount of these sweeteners have been limited to 1 teaspoon or less per serving to ensure the carb count remains low.
- When you see "salt" as an ingredient in the recipes, use pink Himalayan salt or Celtic sea salt. These salts have the most minerals and aren't bleached like traditional table salt.
- Don't forget *food quality*! For these meal plans and the recipes in Part Two of this book, aim for the highest quality you can find (see page 23 for the labels you should be looking for).

A WORD ABOUT SNACKS

When you are in ketosis, your hunger hormones are regulated and you don't experience sudden urges to eat. That being said, when first starting, you may need a few snacks to get you through the transition. Make sure that your snack has at least a tablespoon of healthy fats. Turn to these satisfying recipes when you need a little extra between meals.

- Avocado with extra-virgin olive oil and pink Himalayan salt
- Crudité with Cucumber Tzatziki (page 181)
- Cup of Chicken Bone Broth (page 166) mixed with 1 tablespoon coconut/MCT oil
- Blackberry Coconut Cups (page 88)
- Healing Golden Milk (page 162)

Stocking Your Pantry

For each weekly meal plan that follows, make sure to check out the reference table on pages 34–35 for the pantry items that you will need for the week. These items will be used as ingredients in the delicious Autoimmune Keto meals that you will be cooking, so make sure you have them on hand!

Pantry Staples Checklist

FATS			
	WEEK 1	WEEK 2	WEEK 3
AVOCADO OIL	☐	☐	☐
COCONUT OIL		☐	☐
EXTRA-VIRGIN OLIVE OIL	☐	☐	☐
FULL-FAT COCONUT MILK (KEEP 5 CANS ON HAND)	☐	☐	☐
MCT OIL	☐	☐	☐
UNSWEETENED COCONUT FLAKES		☐	

CONDIMENTS/SAUCES			
	WEEK 1	WEEK 2	WEEK 3
APPLE CIDER VINEGAR	☐	☐	☐
BALSAMIC VINEGAR	☐	☐	☐
CAPERS (1 JAR)	☐	☐	☐
COCONUT AMINOS	☐	☐	☐
FISH SAUCE		☐	☐
PURE VANILLA POWDER			☐
RED WINE VINEGAR	☐	☐	☐

NATURAL SWEETENERS			
	WEEK 1	WEEK 2	WEEK 3
RAW HONEY	☐	☐	☐
PURE MAPLE SYRUP		☐	☐

DRIED SPICES

	WEEK 1	WEEK 2	WEEK 3
BASIL	☐		☐
BAY LEAVES	☐		
CINNAMON	☐	☐	☐
GARLIC POWDER	☐		☐
ONION POWDER	☐		☐
OREGANO	☐	☐	☐
PINK HIMALAYAN SALT/CELTIC SEA SALT	☐	☐	☐
THYME		☐	

POWDERS/TEAS

	WEEK 1	WEEK 2	WEEK 3
BEEF GELATIN POWDER		☐	
COCONUT FLOUR	☐		
COLLAGEN PEPTIDES POWDER	☐	☐	☐
DRIED ROSE PETALS (OPTIONAL)			☐
EARL GREY TEA BAGS			☐
MATCHA POWDER (IDEALLY ORGANIC AND CEREMONIAL GRADE)	☐		

INTERMITTENT FASTING

A powerful technique that works incredibly well with Autoimmune Keto is intermittent fasting. Intermittent fasting is simply a type of eating schedule that gives your body an extended period of time between feedings to digest food and also heal. Intermittent fasting also jump-starts ketosis and promotes autophagy (a fancy word for cellular repair and regeneration).

There are various versions of intermittent fasting methods. Here are the most popular:

- The 16/8 Method - Requires restricting your daily eating period to 8 hours, while fasting for 16 hours in between.
- Eat-Stop-Eat - Requires fasting for 24 hours for 1 or 2 days per week.
- The 5:2 Diet - Requires eating only 500–600 calories on two nonconsecutive days during the week.

When first starting out on Autoimmune Keto, we recommend that you ease into intermittent fasting. A few simple ways to do that can be aiming to stop eating by 7pm each night or waiting until late morning to have your breakfast.

The negative side effect of intermittent fasting is mostly hunger. Most people experience this side effect in the first few days while their body is still adjusting to the method. The key is to listen to your body and check in on how you feel during the fasting periods.

Intermittent fasting is not advised for the following people:

- Anyone struggling with or prone to an eating disorder
- Anyone who has issues with blood sugar regulation
- Anyone who suffers from hypoglycemia or diabetes
- Anyone who is malnourished
- Children under 18 years old
- Pregnant women
- Breastfeeding women
- Anyone taking daily medications that require consumption with food

Week 1

Welcome to the first day of the rest of your life. You are about to embark on a life-changing transformation, and we are so excited for you! This week's meal plan is all about keeping it *simple*. We are going to eat the same breakfast the entire week, as well as leverage weekend meal prep and leftovers.

Shopping List

Organic Produce

FRUITS

- 4 avocados
- 2 lemons

VEGGIES

- 6 asparagus spears
- 6 cups broccoli
- 1 carrot
- 1 head cauliflower
- 2 stalks celery
- 8 cups mixed greens
- 1 large shallot
- 1 yellow onion
- 1 (14-ounce) can hearts of palm
- 1 (14-ounce) can artichoke hearts

FRESH HERBS/SPICES

- 4 garlic bulbs
- 1 bunch cilantro
- 1 bunch parsley

QUALITY PROTEIN

- 8 skinless, boneless chicken thighs
- 4 skin-on chicken thighs
- 1 cod fillet (6 ounces)
- 3 salmon fillets (6 ounces each)
- skirt steak (24 ounces)
- 6 cups Chicken Bone Broth (store-bought or homemade, page 166)

***Make sure to check the **Pantry Staples Checklist** on pages 34–35 to ensure you are properly stocked.

	MEAL 1	MEAL 2	MEAL 3
MONDAY	Creamy Matcha Latte (page 56)	Healing Chicken Soup (page 98)	Skirt Steak with Chimichurri Sauce (page 130) & Broccoli and Shallots (page 79)
TUESDAY	Creamy Matcha Latte (page 56)	Leftover Skirt Steak with Chimichurri Sauce & Broccoli and Shallots	Crispy-Skin Salmon (page 115) & Roasted Garlic Cauliflower Mash (page 76)
WEDNESDAY	Creamy Matcha Latte (page 56)	Leftover Healing Chicken Soup	Artichoke and Hearts of Palm Salad (page 102)
THURSDAY	Creamy Matcha Latte (page 56)	Leftover Artichoke and Hearts of Palm Salad	Crispy-Skin Salmon (page 115) & Leftover Roasted Garlic Cauliflower Mash
FRIDAY	Creamy Matcha Latte (page 56)	Leftover Healing Chicken Soup	Skirt Steak with Chimichurri Sauce (page 130) & Broccoli and Shallots (page 79)
SATURDAY	Creamy Matcha Latte (page 56)	Leftover Skirt Steak with Chimichurri Sauce & Broccoli and Shallots	Crispy-Skin Salmon (page 115) & Leftover Roasted Garlic Cauliflower Mash
SUNDAY	Creamy Matcha Latte (page 56)	Leftover Healing Chicken Soup	Garlic Lemon Cod with Asparagus (page 114)

Weekend Prep Ahead

Below we have outlined the most efficient way to meal prep on the weekend, so that you minimize your time in the kitchen during the week.

Prepare the Vegetables

- Chop the broccoli and cauliflower into florets.
- Peel and chop the carrots into ½-inch pieces.
- Chop the celery into ½-inch pieces.
- Peel and dice the yellow onion.
- Peel and thinly slice the shallot.

- Preheat the oven to 400°F.
- Line a baking sheet with parchment paper.
- Cook the 4 skin-on chicken thighs. Coat the chicken with avocado oil and season with salt. Bake for 20 to 30 minutes or until the juices run clear. Let them cool and store in the refrigerator. You will use these for the Artichoke and Hearts of Palm Salad (page 102) during the week.
- At the same time, roast your garlic cloves for the Roasted Garlic Cauliflower Mash (page 76) at 400°F.
- Prepare the marinade for the Skirt Steak with Chimichurri Sauce (page 130). Add your steak to the marinade and store it in a sealed container in the refrigerator overnight.
- Make the Healing Chicken Soup (page 98). Let the soup cool enough to transfer it to a sealed container and store in the refrigerator. The recipe yields four servings, and you will eat one serving for lunch on Monday, Wednesday, Friday, and Sunday, respectively.
- Make ½ serving of the Autoimmune Keto House Dressing (page 177). Store it in the refrigerator in a sealed container for the Artichoke and Hearts of Palm Salad (page 102) you'll eat this week.
- Make the Chimichurri Sauce (page 175). Store it in the refrigerator in a sealed container for the Skirt Steak with Chimichurri Sauce you'll eat during the week.
- Once the garlic is roasted, make the Roasted Garlic Cauliflower Mash (page 76). Let it cool enough to transfer to a sealed container and store in the refrigerator. The recipe yields three servings and you will eat one serving for dinner on Tuesday, Thursday, and Saturday, respectively.
- At the end of the week on Thursday night, prepare the marinade for the Skirt Steak with Chimichurri Sauce (page 130) one more time. Add your steak to the marinade and store it in a sealed container in the refrigerator overnight.

THE KETO FLU

Keto Flu can occur when your body is transitioning its energy source from glucose to ketones. Symptoms can include headaches, nausea, fatigue, irritability, constipation, and soreness. You'll feel like you have the flu for a few days. Be patient! These symptoms will subside and feeling this way is a good sign that you're getting into ketosis.

To combat keto flu or to attempt to avoid it all together, here are our go-to tips:

Stay Hydrated. Drink at least a half ounce of filtered water for each pound that you weigh. Sprinkle pink Himalayan salt into your water to balance your electrolytes.

Rest. Get plenty of sleep (aim for 7 to 9 hours each night) and don't overdo it with physical activity or exercise.

Up Your Fats. Increase your intake by adding an extra tablespoon of fat to your meal or snacking on high-fat foods like avocados.

Don't worry, the keto flu only lasts 3 to 5 days. Once you get through this transition phase, you begin to reap all the amazing benefits of being in ketosis.

Week 2

Week 2 introduces new meals full of incredible flavors. Once again, this week is AIP-Elimination Phase compliant so all you need to do is follow along. This week changes up the breakfast options, but if you are loving the Creamy Matcha Latte (page 56) from Week 1, feel free to have it instead.

Shopping List

HEALTHY FATS

- 6⅓ cups plain unsweetened Coconut Yogurt (store-bought or homemade, page 178)
- ¼ cup pitted Kalamata olives

Organic Produce

FRUITS

- 2 avocados
- 2 lemons
- 2 limes
- ½ cup raspberries
- 1½ cups frozen strawberries

VEGGIES

- 12 asparagus spears
- 5½ cups baby spinach
- 2 Bibb lettuce leaves
- 2 cups broccoli
- 1 head cauliflower
- 2½ cucumbers
- 1 cup mixed greens
- 4 cups cremini mushrooms
- 1 large red onion
- 1 shallot
- 1 yellow onion

FRESH HERBS/SPICES

- 2 cups basil
- 1 bunch cilantro
- 1 bunch dill
- 4 garlic bulbs
- 1-inch ginger root
- 2-inch piece horseradish
- ¾ cup mint leaves
- 1 bunch parsley
- 2 sprigs fresh thyme

QUALITY PROTEIN

- 4 skin-on chicken thighs
- 1 halibut fillet (6 ounces)
- 10 slices bacon
- 4 slices prosciutto
- 6 ounces scallops
- 6 ounces shrimp
- 1 flank steak (12 ounces)
- 1 skirt steak (12 ounces)
- 8 ounces ground lamb
- ¼ cup Beef Bone Broth (store-bought or homemade, page 168)
- 6 cups Chicken Bone Broth (store-bought or homemade, page 166)

***Make sure to check the **Pantry Staples Checklist** on pages 34–35 to ensure you are properly stocked.

	MEAL 1	MEAL 2	MEAL 3
MONDAY	Coconut Yogurt Berry Parfait (page 63)	Cauliflower and Bacon Soup (page 107)	Greek Meatball Lettuce Wraps (page 133) & Cucumber Herb Salad (page 81)
TUESDAY	Strawberry and Spinach Smoothie (page 60)	Leftover Greek Meatball Lettuce Wraps, Leftover Cucumber Herb Salad	Pesto Halibut in Parchment Paper (page 116) & Sautéed Super Greens (page 80)
WEDNESDAY	Coconut Yogurt Berry Parfait (page 63)	Leftover Cauliflower and Bacon Soup	Flank Steak with Sweet Horseradish Cream (page 135), Garlic and Herb Mushrooms (page 72)
THURSDAY	Strawberry and Spinach Smoothie (page 60)	Leftover Flank Steak with Sweet Horseradish Cream, Leftover Garlic and Herb Mushrooms	Bacon Wrapped Scallops with Sweet Balsamic Sauce (page 110) & Leftover Sautéed Super Greens
FRIDAY	Coconut Yogurt Berry Parfait (page 63)	Leftover Cauliflower and Bacon Soup	Cucumber and Beef Mint Salad (page 103)
SATURDAY	Strawberry and Spinach Smoothie (page 60)	Leftover Cucumber and Beef Mint Salad	Grilled Chicken with Dill Yogurt Sauce (page 122) & Prosciutto-Wrapped Asparagus (page 78)
SUNDAY	Coconut Yogurt Berry Parfait (page 63)	Leftover Grilled Chicken with Dill Yogurt Sauce, Leftover Prosciutto-Wrapped Asparagus	Teriyaki Shrimp and Broccoli (page 112)

Weekend Prep Ahead

Below we have outlined the most efficient way to meal prep on the weekend, so that you minimize your time in the kitchen during the week.

Prepare the Vegetables

- Chop the broccoli and cauliflower into florets.
- Peel and dice the shallot.
- Peel and thinly slice the red onion.
- Peel and dice the yellow onion.

Cook Ahead

- If making homemade Coconut Yogurt (page 178), prepare it (you need to start this on a Saturday morning since it takes 48 hours).
- Make the Coconut Topping (page 63) for the parfaits and store in a sealed container at room temperature.
- Make the Cauliflower and Bacon Soup (page 107). Let the soup cool enough to transfer it to a sealed container and store in the refrigerator. The recipe yields three servings and you will eat one serving for lunch on Monday, Wednesday, and Friday, respectively.
- Make the Greek Meatball Lettuce Wraps (page 133) and store in a sealed container in the refrigerator. Don't assemble the lettuce wraps until you're ready to serve.
- Make the Cucumber Herb Salad (page 81) and store in a sealed container in the refrigerator.
- Make the Basil Pesto (page 174). Store it in the refrigerator in a sealed container for the Pesto Halibut in Parchment Paper (page 116) you'll eat this week.
- Make the Cucumber Tzatziki (page 181). Store it in the refrigerator in a sealed container for the Greek Meatball Lettuce Wraps (page 133) you'll eat this week.
- Make the Sweet Horseradish Cream (page 180). Store it in the refrigerator in a sealed container for the Flank Steak with Sweet Horseradish Cream (page 135) you'll eat this week.
- At the end of the week on either Friday night or Saturday morning, prepare the marinade for the Grilled Chicken with Dill Yogurt Sauce (page 122). Add your skin-on chicken thighs to the marinade and store it in a sealed container in the refrigerator for 3 to 5 hours during the day.

Week 3

You are on Week 3 already! This week is still AIP-Elimination Phase compliant, so once again all you need to do is follow along. By now, you should be in ketosis and burning ketones as fuel!

Shopping List

HEALTHY FATS

- ⅔ cup plain unsweetened Coconut Yogurt (store-bought or home-made, page 178)
- ¼ cup pitted Kalamata olives

Organic Produce

FRUITS

- 4 avocados
- 3 lemons
- 4 limes
- ¾ cup pumpkin purée
- 1 large grapefruit (need 1 cup fresh juice)

VEGGIES

- 6 asparagus spears
- 4 cups baby spinach
- 3 cups broccoli
- 1 head cauliflower
- 8 cups mixed greens
- 1 large red onion
- 6 cups romaine
- 1 shallot
- 1 cup white button mushrooms
- 1 (14 ounce) can hearts of palm
- 1 (14 ounce) can artichoke hearts

FRESH HERBS/SPICES

- 2 cups basil leaves
- 1 small bunch cilantro
- 1 bunch dill
- 4 garlic bulbs
- 1-inch piece ginger root
- 1 stalk lemongrass
- 1 bunch parsley

QUALITY PROTEIN

- 8 skin-on chicken thighs
- 4 skinless, boneless chicken thighs
- 1 cod fillet (6 ounces)
- 8 ounces ground beef
- 1 halibut fillet (6 ounces)
- 4 slices bacon
- 1 salmon fillet (6 ounces)
- 6 ounces scallops
- 1 skirt steak (12 ounces)

***Make sure to check the **Pantry Staples Checklist** on pages 34–35 to ensure you are properly stocked.

	MEAL 1	MEAL 2	MEAL 3
MONDAY	Earl Grey Rose Latte (page 58)	Artichoke and Hearts of Palm Salad (page 102)	Bacon-Wrapped Scallops with Sweet Balsamic Sauce (page 110) & Broccoli and Shallots (page 79)
TUESDAY	Pumpkin Breakfast Smoothie (page 61)	Tom Kha Gai (page 100)	Skirt Steak with Chimichurri Sauce (page 130) & Roasted Garlic Cauliflower Mash (page 76)
WEDNESDAY	Earl Grey Rose Latte (page 58)	Leftover Skirt Steak with Chimichurri Sauce, Leftover Roasted Garlic Cauliflower Mash	Crispy-Skin Salmon (page 115) & Leftover Broccoli and Shallots
THURSDAY	Pumpkin Breakfast Smoothie (page 61)	Leftover Tom Kha Gai	Cilantro Lime Taco Bowls (page 134)
FRIDAY	Earl Grey Rose Latte (page 58)	Leftover Cilantro Lime Taco Bowls	Grilled Chicken with Dill Yogurt Sauce (page 122) & Sautéed Super Greens (page 80)
SATURDAY	Pumpkin Breakfast Smoothie (page 61)	Leftover Grilled Chicken with Dill Yogurt Sauce & Leftover Sautéed Super Greens	Garlic Lemon Cod with Asparagus (page 114)
SUNDAY	Earl Grey Rose Latte (page 58)	Leftover Artichoke and Hearts of Palm Salad	Pesto Halibut in Parchment Paper (page 116) & Leftover Roasted Garlic Cauliflower Mash

Weekend Prep Ahead

Below we have outlined the most efficient way to meal prep on the weekend, so that you minimize your time in the kitchen during the week.

Prepare the Vegetables

- Chop the broccoli and cauliflower into florets.
- Peel and dice the red onion.
- Peel and thinly slice the shallot.

- Preheat the oven to 400°F.
- Line a baking sheet with parchment paper.
- Cook 4 of the skin-on chicken thighs. Coat the chicken with avocado oil and season with salt. Bake for 20 to 30 minutes or until juices run clear. Let them cool and store in the refrigerator. You will use these for the Artichoke and Hearts of Palm Salad (page 102) you'll eat this week.
- At the same time, roast your garlic cloves for the Roasted Garlic Cauliflower Mash (page 76) at 400°F for 40 to 45 minutes.
- Prepare your marinade for the Skirt Steak with Chimichurri Sauce (page 130). Add your steak to the marinade and store it in a sealed container in the refrigerator. You will grill this steak on Tuesday night.
- Make the Tom Kha Gai (page 100). Let the soup cool enough to transfer it to a sealed container and store in the refrigerator. The recipe yields 2 servings and you will eat one serving for lunch on Tuesday and Thursday, respectively.
- Make a half serving of the Autoimmune Keto House Dressing (page 177). Store it in the refrigerator in a sealed container for the Artichoke and Hearts of Palm Salad (page 102) you'll eat this week.
- Make the Chimichurri Sauce. Store it in the refrigerator in a sealed container for the Skirt Steak with Chimichurri Sauce you'll eat this week.
- Make the Basil Pesto (page 174). Store it in the refrigerator in a sealed container for the Pesto Halibut in Parchment Paper (page 116) you'll eat this week.
- Make the Grapefruit Red Onions (page 182) for the Cilantro Lime Taco Bowls (page 134) you'll eat this week. Store them in a large mason jar in the refrigerator.
- Once the garlic is roasted, make the Roasted Garlic Cauliflower Mash (page 76).
- On Thursday night, prepare the marinade for the Grilled Chicken with Dill Yogurt Sauce (page 122). Add your remaining 4 skin-on chicken thighs to the marinade and store them in a sealed container in the refrigerator overnight.

How to Build Your Own Meal Plan

Going forward, feel free to repeat any of these weekly meal plans. We also encourage you to build your own meal plans using our 8-3-6 Formula that we discussed earlier in the book on page 27. Aim to have at least two servings of fat at each meal to keep you satiated and energized.

Part Two of this book is dedicated entirely to recipes and to make it even easier, we have clearly labeled each recipe either AIP-Elimination Phase or AIP-Reintroduction Phase. In addition, we have added the label "Super Quick" to any recipes that take 30 minutes or less to prepare. Use these recipes as inspiration for your weekly meal plans.

The Reintroduction Phase

Autoimmune Keto isn't designed for you to stay in the Elimination Phase for the rest of your life. Once you start feeling well and your autoimmune symptoms have dissipated, it is time for the Reintroduction Phase!

There is no set timeframe for how long you should stay in the Elimination Phase. It really depends on the person, but we highly recommend staying in the Elimination Phase for a minimum of 5 weeks before reintroducing any new foods. In general, most of our clients start the Reintroduction Phase between 5 and 12 weeks after beginning the Elimination Phase. Listen to your body and pay attention to its signals such as cravings for certain type of foods or your intuition telling you that it is ready to reintroduce a food category. You will know when it is time.

The key to the Reintroduction Phase is doing it strategically in stages. The goal is to slowly add in certain foods in a specific order and then allow sufficient time to see how your body reacts to those foods. It's really important during this phase to track everything so you can make an informed decision on what works and what doesn't for your body. We have added a Reintroduction Phase Worksheet on page 49 to help facilitate this tracking.

Reintroduction Stages

We organized the Reintroduction Phase into 5 distinct stages. These stages are based on our own experience and what worked best for us.

STAGE	FOODS TO REINTRODUCE
1	NON-AIP SPICES AND GHEE
2	EGGS & EGG-BASED SAUCES
3	SEEDS, NUTS, AND BUTTER
4	NIGHTSHADES AND OTHER DAIRY
5	LOW-SUGAR ALCOHOL & KETO SWEETENERS

The categories detailed in the stages above line up with the *Foods to Avoid Initially but Can Be Reintroduced* list on page 25, so you can see exactly what foods are in that category. Any food item that is not considered keto and is listed on *Foods To Avoid* on page 26, will not be on this list because at the end of the day, we want you to continue living in ketosis long-term! By the end of these five stages, you will have a customized list of foods you can eat that are tailored to your body's needs! How incredible is that?

How to Reintroduce Foods

When reintroducing foods, you need to take a measured approach. First, start with just **one** bite, slowly chew it, and then swallow. Wait 20 minutes and see if you experience any immediate reactions. If there are no reactions, have a few more bites. Again, wait 20 minutes for any reactions or symptoms. If there are still no reactions, eat another few bites. This time, wait three hours for any reactions or symptoms to appear. If you still don't have any, eat a normal quantity of the food and monitor for the next seven days.

During this seven-day period, don't reintroduce any other foods and pay attention to body signals like fatigue, digestive distress, headaches, poor sleep, joint pain, skin irritations, or mood changes, and check if any of your autoimmune symptoms resurface. If after seven days, you still have no reactions or symptoms, you can reintroduce this food permanently into your diet. If at any time during this process, you do experience a negative reaction or notice symptoms, mark this food as a "No" for reintroduction at this time.

If you have a really bad reaction to a food that doesn't subside, go back to the Elimination Phase before proceeding further. Remember, this is a journey, not a race! Take your time with the Reintroduction Phase.

Reintroduction Phase Worksheet: Tracking What Works for You

NAME OF FOOD	DATE & TIME	INITIAL REACTION	3 HOUR REACTION	7 DAY SYMPTOMS	REINTRODUCE (YES OR NO)
Eggplant					
Peppers (all kinds)					
Tomatillos					
Tomatoes					
Butter					
Buttermilk					
Cheese					
Ghee					
Full-fat yogurt					
Heavy cream					
Sour cream					
Whey					
Aioli					
Béarnaise					
Eggs					
Mayonnaise					

CONTINUED

NAME OF FOOD	DATE & TIME	INITIAL REACTION	3 HOUR REACTION	7 DAY SYMPTOMS	REINTRODUCE (YES OR NO)
Almonds					
Brazil nuts					
Cashews					
Macadamia nuts					
Pecans					
Pine nuts					
Pistachios					
Walnuts					
Cacao					
Chia seeds					
Cocoa					
Coffee					
Flax seeds					
Hemp seeds					
Poppy seeds					
Pumpkin seeds					
Sesame seeds					
Sunflower seeds					

NAME OF FOOD	DATE & TIME	INITIAL REACTION	3 HOUR REACTION	7 DAY SYMPTOMS	REINTRODUCE (YES OR NO)
Allspice					
Anise					
Black/white pepper					
Caraway					
Cardamom					
Celery seed					
Coriander					
Cumin					
Dill seed					
Fennel seed					
Juniper					
Mustard seed					
Nutmeg					
Erythritol					
Monk fruit extract					
Stevia					
Clear liquors					
Dry wines					

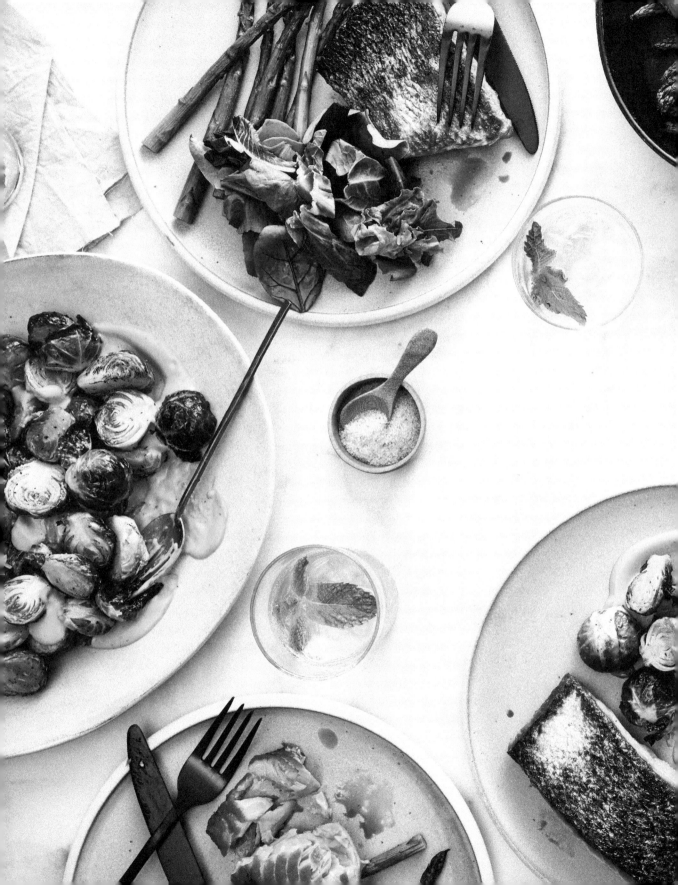

PART TWO

THE AUTOIMMUNE
KETO RECIPES

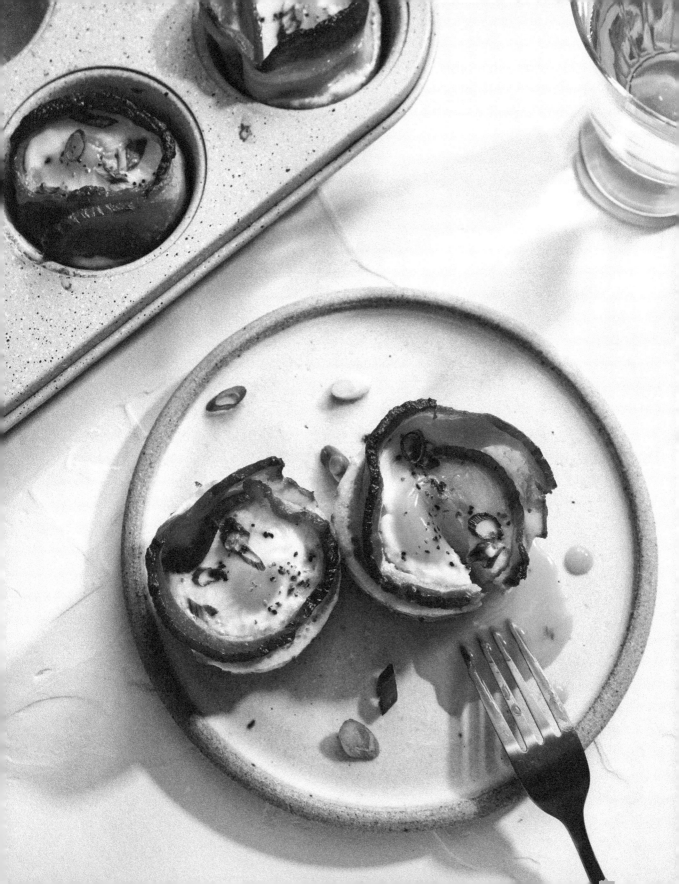

Chapter 3

BREAKFAST

CREAMY MATCHA LATTE

PREP TIME: 5 MINUTES | COOK TIME: 5 MINUTES

AIP-Elimination Phase Compliant

SERVES 1

This Creamy Matcha Latte is the perfect coffee replacement during the Elimination Phase of AIP. Packed with natural energy from the matcha powder and healthy fats to keep you fueled, this breakfast beverage is a great way to jumpstart your day. Matcha is also full of antioxidants, including EGCG (epigallocatechin gallate), which is thought to reduce inflammation, and is also rich in fiber, chlorophyll, and other vitamins.

1 teaspoon matcha powder

⅓ cup hot filtered water
   (not boiling)

1½ cups full-fat
   coconut milk

1 tablespoon collagen
   peptides powder

1 teaspoon MCT oil

1 teaspoon raw
   honey (optional)

Ground cinnamon,
   for garnish

1. Place the matcha powder in a small bowl. Pour in the hot filtered water. Using a spoon or a bamboo whisk, stir until well combined with no visible clumps.

2. Meanwhile, heat the coconut milk in a saucepan over medium heat until it comes to a light simmer. Once simmering, remove the saucepan from heat and stir in the matcha mixture.

3. Transfer the coconut matcha mixture to a blender and add in the collagen, MCT oil, and honey (if using).

4. Blend for 10 to 30 seconds or until fully combined. *(The liquids will be hot, so put a dish towel over the opening of the blender before turning it on.)*

5. Pour the matcha latte into a large mug and sprinkle with cinnamon. Serve immediately.

Tip: Be sure to use full-fat coconut milk with no additives. The only ingredients should be coconut and water. We like Native Forest Simple Coconut Milk, which comes in a can. Also, make sure to shake the can vigorously before opening to combine the coconut and water.

Swap: To lower the carb content, you can swap out the honey for 1 teaspoon of erythritol or 4 drops liquid stevia extract if these have been successfully reintroduced.

Per Serving Calories: 674; Total Fat: 62g; Total Carbs: 13g; Fiber: 5g; Net Carbs: 8g; Protein: 16g MACROS - Fat: 83%; Protein: 9%; Carbs: 8%

EARL GREY ROSE LATTE

PREP TIME: 5 MINUTES | COOK TIME: 5 MINUTES

AIP-Elimination Phase Compliant

SERVES 1

Earl Grey tea contains bergamot oil, a powerful polyphenol that is known for its natural healing properties and for promoting cellular regeneration. This latte is incredibly rich and creamy, plus it will keep you satisfied and energized all morning long.

1 cup filtered water

1 Earl Grey tea bag (make sure the only ingredients are black tea and bergamot oil)

1 tablespoon dried rose petals (optional)

1 cup full-fat coconut milk

1 tablespoon collagen peptide powder

1 teaspoon MCT oil

1 teaspoon raw honey (optional)

1. Bring the water to a boil in a kettle or saucepan over high heat. Pour the boiling water into a large mug or teapot.

2. Add the tea bag and dried rose petals (if using) to the water and allow to steep for 4 to 5 minutes.

3. Meanwhile, heat the coconut milk in a saucepan over medium heat until it comes to a light simmer.

4. Once simmering, remove the saucepan from heat and transfer the coconut milk to a blender. Add in the collagen, MCT oil, and honey (if using).

5. Using a mesh strainer, pour the tea into the blender.

6. Blend for 10 to 30 seconds or until fully combined. *(The liquids will be hot, so put a dish towel over the opening of the blender before turning it on.)*

7. Pour the latte mixture into a large mug and serve.

Tip: Rose petals are a fabulous way to add aroma and flavor to any drink. You can buy dried rose petals on Amazon or at stores such as World Market.

Swap: To lower the carb content, you can swap out the honey for 1 teaspoon of erythritol or 4 drops liquid stevia extract if these have been successfully reintroduced.

Per Serving Calories: 661; Total Fat: 62g; Total Carbs: 13g; Fiber: 5g; Net Carbs: 8g; Protein: 15g MACROS - Fat: 83%; Protein: 9%; Carbs: 8%

STRAWBERRY AND SPINACH SMOOTHIE

PREP TIME: 5 MINUTES

AIP-Elimination Phase Compliant

SERVES 1

Spinach is loaded with vitamins and minerals including iron, magnesium, calcium, folic acid, calcium, vitamins B6 and B9, and antioxidants. It also has a very mild taste, which makes it a perfect choice to add a nutrient boost to a smoothie!

1 cup full-fat coconut milk
½ cup frozen strawberries
½ cup baby spinach
1 tablespoon collagen
  peptides powder
1 teaspoon MCT oil
1 cup ice

Place all the ingredients into a blender, and process until smooth. Pour into a glass and serve.

Tips: For a thicker smoothie, add ½ cup frozen cauliflower. It is flavorless, but adds a creamy texture along with extra vegetables. You can make this smoothie ahead of time and refrigerate it in a mason jar for up to 3 days.

Per Serving: Calories: 589; Total Fat: 54g; Total Carbs: 9g; Fiber: 2g; Net Carbs: 7g; Protein: 12g MACROS - Fat: 83%; Protein: 9%; Carbs: 8%

PUMPKIN BREAKFAST SMOOTHIE

PREP TIME: 5 MINUTES

AIP-Elimination Phase Compliant

SERVES 1

Pumpkin contains beta-carotene, a powerful antioxidant that is converted by the body into vitamin A. It is also rich in fiber, potassium, and vitamin C. For an easy on-the-go breakfast, make this pumpkin and coconut milk–based smoothie. Just throw everything into a blender and you will have a super delicious breakfast in no time!

1 cup full-fat coconut milk

¼ cup pumpkin purée

1 tablespoon collagen peptides powder

½ teaspoon ground cinnamon

½ teaspoon vanilla powder

1 teaspoon MCT oil

1 teaspoon pure maple syrup (optional)

1 cup ice

Pour the coconut milk, pumpkin purée, collagen powder, cinnamon, vanilla powder, MCT oil, maple syrup (if using), and ice into a blender, then process until smooth. Pour into a glass and serve.

Tip: During the Elimination Phase of AIP, avoid using vanilla extract in raw foods where the alcohol will not cook off. Instead, opt for pure vanilla powder, which you can find online or at most health food stores.

Swap: To lower the carb content, you can swap out the pure maple syrup for 1 teaspoon of erythritol or 4 drops liquid stevia extract if these have been successfully reintroduced.

Per Serving: Calories: 562; Total Fat: 53g; Total Carbs: 11g; Fiber: 2g; Net Carbs: 9g; Protein: 11g MACROS · Fat: 85%; Protein: 8%; Carbs: 7%

AVOCADO AND SMOKED SALMON STACK WITH DILL CAPER SAUCE

PREP TIME: 5 MINUTES

AIP-Elimination Phase Compliant

SERVES 1

When you are in the mood for something clean, fresh, and loaded with healthy fats, make this breakfast dish. This quick meal is full of rich, herby, and tangy flavors that will keep you feeling satiated all morning long.

2 ounces smoked salmon

1 tablespoon extra-virgin olive oil

½ avocado, sliced

¼ cup cucumber, diced

FOR THE DILL CAPER SAUCE

2 tablespoons plain unsweetened Coconut Yogurt (page 178)

2 tablespoons chopped fresh dill

1 teaspoon chopped capers

¼ teaspoon caper juice

¼ teaspoon lemon juice

1. Set the salmon on a plate and top with the olive oil, avocado, and cucumber.

2. In a small bowl, mix together the coconut yogurt, dill, capers, caper juice, and lemon juice until well combined.

3. Top the salmon stack with the Dill Caper Sauce and serve.

Tip: If you don't have time to make the homemade Coconut Yogurt on page 178, feel free to use a store-bought version. Just make sure the only ingredients on the food label are coconut, water, and probiotic cultures. We like the brands Anita's and GT's CocoYo.

Swaps: If you have successfully reintroduced dairy, you can substitute 2 tablespoons of sour cream or crème fraîche for the coconut yogurt in the Dill Caper Sauce. If you have successfully reintroduced eggs, you can add soft or hard-boiled eggs to the dish.

Per Serving: Calories: 411; Total Fat: 35g; Total Carbs: 10g; Fiber: 6g; Net Carbs: 4g; Protein: 14g MACROS · Fat: 77%; Protein: 13%; Carbs: 10%

COCONUT YOGURT BERRY PARFAIT

PREP TIME: 5 MINUTES | COOK TIME: 25 MINUTES

AIP-Elimination Phase Compliant

SERVES 1

This coconut parfait is an easy make-ahead breakfast. Prepare the coconut topping over the weekend and store it in a sealed container for use throughout the week. It is great to have on hand to sprinkle into smoothies and add some crunch to salads.

FOR THE COCONUT TOPPING (MAKES 4 SERVINGS)

½ teaspoon ground cinnamon

½ teaspoon raw honey

½ teaspoon filtered water

½ cup unsweetened coconut flakes

TO MAKE THE COCONUT TOPPING

1. Preheat the oven to 300°F. Line a baking sheet with parchment paper.

2. In a small bowl, combine the cinnamon, honey, and water.

3. Carefully stir in the dried coconut flakes until they are fully coated.

4. Pour the coconut flakes onto the baking sheet and spread them out into an even layer.

5. Bake for 15 to 20 minutes or until the coconut flakes turn golden, stirring halfway.

6. Let the coconut flakes cool completely before transferring to a sealed container. Store in the refrigerator for up to a week.

CONTINUED

FOR THE PARFAIT (MAKES 1 SERVING)

1 cup plain unsweetened Coconut Yogurt (page 178)

1 teaspoon MCT oil

2 tablespoons Coconut Topping

2 tablespoons fresh raspberries

TO MAKE THE PARFAIT

1. Scoop the coconut yogurt into a bowl and stir in the MCT oil.

2. Top the yogurt with the Coconut Topping and raspberries.

Tip: If you don't have time to make the homemade Coconut Yogurt on page 178, feel free to use a store-bought version. Just make sure the only ingredients on the food label are coconut, water, and probiotic cultures. We like the brands Anita's and GT's CocoYo.

Swap: If you have successfully reintroduced nuts, you can add macadamia nuts, walnuts, or pecans to this parfait for some extra crunch and healthy fats!

Per Serving: Calories: 665; Total Fat: 65g; Total Carbs: 12g; Fiber: 3g; Net Carbs: 9g; Protein: 8g MACROS - Fat: 88%; Protein: 5%; Carbs: 7%

BISCUITS WITH SAUSAGE GRAVY

PREP TIME: 10 MINUTES | COOK TIME: 20 MINUTES

AIP-Elimination Phase Compliant

SERVES 4

For a hearty breakfast that you can whip up quickly, make these AIP-Elimination Phase Compliant biscuits with sausage gravy. Make sure to use frozen coconut oil so that it doesn't melt when you are making the dough, and also to create a denser biscuit.

FOR THE BISCUITS

¼ cup frozen coconut oil

½ cup, plus 2 tablespoons coconut flour

6 tablespoons plain unsweetened Coconut Yogurt (page 178)

2 teaspoons apple cider vinegar

1 tablespoon, plus 1 teaspoon baking powder

½ teaspoon salt

½ teaspoon garlic powder

½ teaspoon onion powder

1 tablespoon melted coconut oil

TO MAKE THE BISCUITS

1. Preheat the oven to 450°F. Line a baking sheet with parchment paper.

2. Chop the frozen coconut oil into very small pieces.

3. In a medium bowl, mix together the coconut flour, coconut yogurt, apple cider vinegar, baking powder, salt, garlic powder, and onion powder.

4. Add the frozen coconut oil pieces to the flour mixture. Work the dough with your hands and break apart any solid coconut oil pieces.

5. Form the dough into six biscuit shapes, packing the dough together lightly. Arrange them on the baking sheet.

6. Brush the melted coconut oil on top of each biscuit.

7. Bake for 10 minutes or until golden brown.

CONTINUED

FOR THE SAUSAGE GRAVY

1 pound ground pork

2 teaspoons fresh sage

1 teaspoon salt

1 teaspoon fresh thyme

½ teaspoon garlic powder

¼ teaspoon onion powder

1 tablespoon coconut flour

1 cup full-fat coconut milk

TO MAKE THE SAUSAGE GRAVY

1. Combine the ground pork and spices in a bowl.

2. Heat a large skillet over medium heat and brown the sausage.

3. Once the sausage is cooked through, add in the coconut flour and cook for 2 more minutes.

4. Stir in the coconut milk and let the gravy cook for an additional 5 to 10 minutes.

5. Serve over the biscuits.

Tip: If you don't have time to make the homemade Coconut Yogurt on page 178, feel free to use a store-bought version. Just make sure the only ingredients on the food label are coconut, water, and probiotic cultures. We like the brands Anita's and GT's CocoYo.

Swap: You can substitute ghee or grass-fed butter for the coconut oil if these have been successfully reintroduced.

Per Serving Calories: 722; Total Fat: 62g; Total Carbs: 17g; Fiber: 8g; Net Carbs: 9g; Protein: 24g MACROS - Fat: 77%; Protein: 14%; Carbs: 9%

BACON-WRAPPED EGG CUPS

PREP TIME: 10 MINUTES | COOK TIME: 20 MINUTES

AIP-Reintroduction Phase: Eggs & Egg-Based Sauces,
Non-AIP Spices (black pepper)

SERVES 3 (MAKES 6 EGG CUPS)

This super low-carb breakfast is easy to make in a muffin pan and has a fun presentation. Add avocado slices or fresh herbs to the tops of the cooked egg cups to take them up a notch.

6 slices bacon (nitrate-free, no sugar added)

1 teaspoon avocado oil

6 large eggs

2 tablespoons chopped scallions

¼ teaspoon salt

⅛ teaspoon black pepper

1. Preheat the oven to 375°F. Line a baking sheet with parchment paper.

2. Add the bacon to the baking sheet and cook for 6 minutes in the oven. Remove the bacon from the oven and let cool slightly.

3. Grease a six-cup muffin pan with the avocado oil.

4. Carefully place each bacon slice inside the muffin cup creating a circle around the edge of each well.

5. Crack one egg into each muffin cup; top with the scallions, salt, and pepper.

6. Bake for 12 to 14 minutes, until the egg white is cooked but the yolk is still runny.

7. Let cool for 1 to 2 minutes then remove each egg cup carefully with a spoon and serve.

Tip: Using a thicker cut of bacon will result in a sturdier egg cup. Look for bacon that doesn't contain nitrates or added sugar.

Per Serving: Calories: 244; Total Fat: 18g; Total Carbs: 1g; Fiber: 0g; Net Carbs: 1g; Protein: 19g MACROS - Fat: 67%; Protein: 31%; Carbs: 2%

CHESAPEAKE EGGS BENEDICT

PREP TIME: 5 MINUTES | COOK TIME: 25 MINUTES

AIP-Reintroduction Phase: Dairy (ghee), Eggs & Egg-Based Sauces, Nightshades (cayenne), Non-AIP Spices (Seafood Seasoning)

SERVES 2

We gave this classic breakfast dish a low-carb makeover by ditching the English muffin and using a bed of roasted asparagus instead. The crab meat and poached eggs complement each other beautifully, and you can't go wrong with a rich hollandaise sauce that ties the whole plate together.

1 pound asparagus, woody ends removed

2 tablespoons avocado oil

¼ teaspoon salt

8 ounces lump crab meat

1 tablespoon avocado-oil based mayonnaise (like Primal Kitchen brand)

⅛ teaspoon Seafood Seasoning (page 183)

4 eggs

1 tablespoon apple cider vinegar

1 tablespoon fresh parsley, chopped, for garnish (optional)

TO MAKE THE EGGS BENEDICT

1. Preheat the oven to 400°F.

2. Place the trimmed asparagus on a baking sheet and toss with the avocado oil and salt.

3. Bake for 8 to 10 minutes, turn off the oven, and keep the asparagus warmed inside as you make the crab mixture and eggs.

4. In a medium bowl, gently fold together the crab meat, mayonnaise, and seasoning. Set aside.

5. Prepare the poached eggs by bringing a large pot of filtered water to a boil. Stir in the vinegar and reduce the heat so that the water is at a simmer.

6. Crack each egg into a ramekin, then gently place the egg into the water. Do not stir.

7. Let the eggs poach for 4 to 5 minutes, then remove them with a slotted spoon. Place the eggs on a separate plate.

8. Assemble your dish by first plating the asparagus, then crab mixture on top, followed by the poached eggs, and lastly the Hollandaise Sauce.

9. Garnish with a generous sprinkle of Seafood Seasoning and parsley.

FOR THE HOLLANDAISE SAUCE

2 egg yolks

1½ tablespoons lemon juice

¼ cup ghee

Light sprinkle of salt

Light dash of cayenne
    pepper

TO MAKE THE HOLLANDAISE SAUCE

1. Fill a small pot with 1 to 2 inches of water. Place a shallow glass or metal bowl inside the pot. The bowl should not be touching the water. (Alternately, you can use a double boiler if you have one.)

2. Heat the pot over medium heat to bring the water to a simmer.

3. In your glass or metal bowl, whisk the yolks and lemon juice together vigorously for 2 minutes.

4. In separate saucepan, melt the ghee. Slowly pour the melted ghee into the yolk mixture, whisking vigorously for another 1 to 2 minutes.

5. When your sauce begins to thicken, turn off the heat and add the salt and cayenne.

Tip: Hollandaise can seize up if the yolks are overcooked, causing your sauce to become too thick. To avoid this, watch your sauce carefully and remove it from the heat once you notice it start to thicken. If it does thicken too much, thin it out by whisking in a teaspoon or two of water.

Per Serving Calories: 756; Total Fat: 60g; Total Carbs: 13g; Fiber: 5g; Net Carbs: 8g; Protein: 45g MACROS - Fat: 70%; Protein: 24%; Carbs: 6%

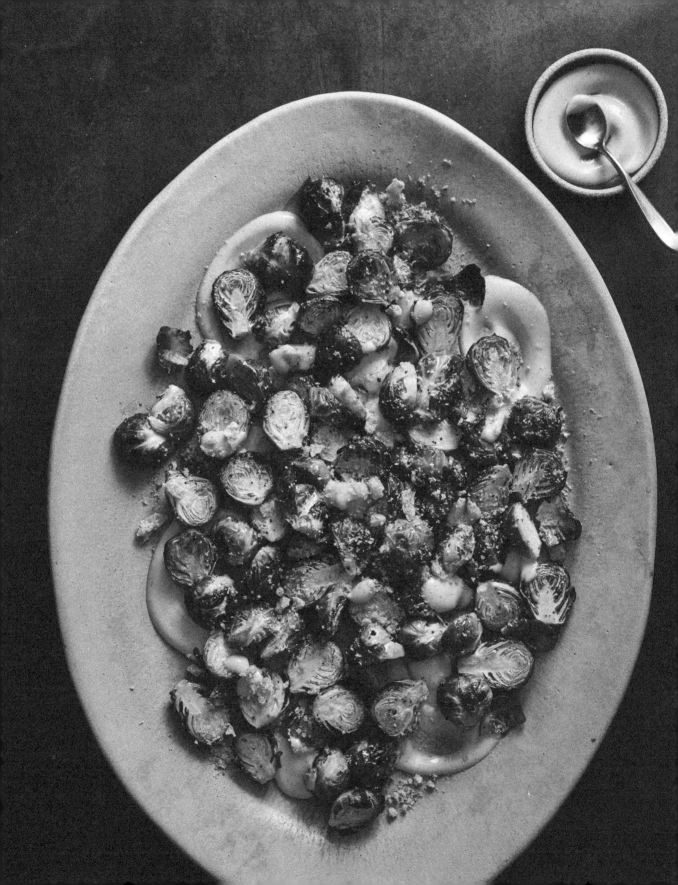

Chapter 4

SIDES

GARLIC AND HERB MUSHROOMS

PREP TIME: 5 MINUTES | COOK TIME: 20 MINUTES

AIP-Elimination Phase Compliant

SERVES 2

Cremini mushrooms are rich in B vitamins, calcium, iron, selenium, and antioxidants, making them a perfect addition to an anti-inflammatory diet. This earthy and herby dish is completely AIP-Elimination Phase compliant, making it one of our favorite healthy sides to serve! It is so fast and easy to prepare, you will want to make it again and again.

1 tablespoon chopped fresh thyme

2 cloves garlic, minced

2 tablespoons avocado oil

4 cups whole cremini mushrooms, dirt wiped away with damp towel

1 teaspoon lemon juice

½ teaspoon salt

1. Preheat the oven to 375°F. Line a baking sheet with parchment paper.

2. In a large bowl, stir the thyme and garlic into the avocado oil. Add the mushrooms.

3. Spread the mushrooms in a single layer on the baking sheet.

4. Pour the lemon juice over the mushrooms.

5. Sprinkle the mushrooms with salt.

6. Bake for 15 to 20 minutes, until browned.

Swap: You can substitute the avocado oil for ghee or grass-fed butter if these have been successfully reintroduced.

Per Serving Calories: 168; Total Fat: 14g; Total Carbs: 7g; Fiber: 1g; Net Carbs: 6g; Protein: 4g MACROS · Fat: 74%; Protein: 9%; Carbs: 17%

STEAMED ARTICHOKES WITH BALSAMIC DIPPING SAUCE

PREP TIME: 10 MINUTES | COOK TIME: 30 MINUTES

AIP-Elimination Phase Compliant

SERVES 4

The artichoke's active ingredient, cynarin, has been proven to aid in digestion and even has been shown to significantly improve IBS symptoms. It also has anti-oxidants, which make this wonderful vegetable perfect for anyone suffering from autoimmune diseases.

Juice from ½ lemon

1 tablespoon salt, plus a pinch for the dipping sauce

4 artichokes

¼ cup balsamic vinegar

¼ cup extra-virgin olive oil

1. In a large pot filled with 1 inch of filtered water, add in the lemon juice and 1 tablespoon of salt, and insert a steamer basket.

2. Prepare the artichokes. Pull off the tough outer leaves and use a sharp serrated knife to cut off the top third of each artichoke. Trim the stems. Use kitchen shears to trim any thorny leaf tips.

3. Place the artichokes in the steamer basket, stem-side up. Cover with a lid and steam about 30 minutes, until the artichoke heart is tender.

4. In a small bowl, combine the balsamic vinegar, olive oil, and a pinch of salt.

5. Pour the dipping sauce into a small dish and serve with the steamed artichokes.

Tip: To prevent your artichokes from discoloring, rub the surface of the artichokes with lemon juice.

Per Serving Calories: 195; Total Fat: 14g; Total Carbs: 17g; Fiber: 7g; Net Carbs: 10g; Protein: 4g MACROS - Fat: 62%; Protein: 5%; Carbs: 33%

CAULIFLOWER ZUCCHINI AND BACON GRATIN

PREP TIME: 25 MINUTES | COOK TIME: 45 MINUTES

AIP-Elimination Phase Compliant

SERVES 8

You'll never believe this gratin has no cheese and is completely AIP compliant! This dish has tender zucchini and cauliflower with a lick-the-plate delicious "cheese" sauce coating every bite. The sauce is extremely versatile: You can also use it over sautéed broccoli or to make a "cheesy" chicken casserole.

8 slices bacon (nitrate-free, no sugar added)

2 heads (about 8 cups) cauliflower, chopped into large florets, divided

4 cloves garlic

1 cup full-fat coconut milk

½ cup Chicken Bone Broth (store-bought or homemade, page 166)

1 tablespoon fish sauce (like Red Boat brand)

1 tablespoon apple cider vinegar

Pinch salt

1 large zucchini, cut into slices

1 tablespoon fresh parsley, chopped, for garnish (optional)

1. Preheat the oven to 350°F.

2. In a large skillet, cook the bacon over medium heat for 10 to 12 minutes, or until crisped. Transfer the bacon to a paper towel-lined plate. Reserve ¼ cup of the bacon fat.

3. In a large pot filled with one inch of filtered water, insert a steamer basket. Place half of the cauliflower florets in the steamer basket. Cover with a lid and bring to a boil. Steam for 10 minutes or until tender.

4. Place the steamed cauliflower, garlic cloves, coconut milk, bone broth, reserved bacon fat, fish sauce, vinegar, and salt in a food processor or blender. Process for about 5 minutes or until a smooth "cheesy" sauce forms.

5. In the same steamer pot, add in the other half of the cauli-flower florets. Cover with a lid, bring to a boil, and steam for 5 minutes.

6. While the cauliflower is steaming, coarsely chop the bacon slices into ½-inch pieces.

7. In an 8-by-11-inch casserole dish, arrange the just steamed cauliflower pieces, zucchini slices, and half of the bacon pieces.

8. Next, pour the "cheese" sauce into the casserole dish and then top with the remaining bacon pieces.

9. Bake for 30 minutes.

10. Remove from oven and garnish with parsley.

Tip: This recipe yields 8 servings, so you will most likely have leftovers. Store them in a sealed container in the refrigerator for up to 3 days. Also, make sure to check the ingredients on the bacon package and ensure that any added spices are AIP-friendly.

Per Serving Calories: 138; Total Fat: 10g; Total Carbs: 9g; Fiber: 4g; Net Carbs: 5g; Protein: 7g MACROS - Fat: 60%; Protein: 16%; Carbs: 24%

ROASTED GARLIC CAULIFLOWER MASH

PREP TIME: 10 MINUTES | COOK TIME: 1 HOUR

AIP-Elimination Phase Compliant

SERVES 3

Cauliflower is so versatile and makes a terrific keto and AIP-friendly substitute for traditional mashed potatoes. We added roasted garlic to take this recipe to another level! Roasting garlic brings out a deeper flavor with hints of sweetness and caramel, making it a perfect addition to this side dish.

1 head garlic

1 tablespoon avocado oil

1 head (about 4 cups) cauliflower, chopped into large florets

¼ cup extra-virgin olive oil

½ teaspoon salt

1 tablespoon fresh parsley, chopped, for garnish (optional)

1. Preheat the oven to 400°F.

2. Slice off the top of the garlic bulb and drizzle avocado oil over the exposed cloves.

3. Wrap the garlic head in parchment paper and then wrap with aluminum foil. Make sure the parchment is not directly touching the exposed cloves.

4. Place the garlic in the oven and roast for 40 to 45 minutes or until soft. Remove from the oven and let cool.

5. As the garlic cools, fill a large pot with one inch of filtered water, insert a steamer basket and place the cauliflower florets in the steamer basket. Cover with a lid and bring to a boil. Steam for 10 minutes or until tender.

6. Transfer the steamed cauliflower to a food processor or blender and squeeze in the individual cloves of roasted garlic.

7. Add in the olive oil and process the cauliflower mixture for 2 minutes or until smooth.

8. Season with salt to taste, drizzle with additional olive oil, and garnish with parsley.

Tip: Roast 2 to 3 garlic bulbs at a time. Let them cool completely and then peel the individual garlic cloves. Place the peeled cloves in a small jar and cover completely with extra-virgin olive oil. Seal the jar and store in the refrigerator for up to 2 weeks to use in sauces and dressings.

Per Serving Calories: 266; Total Fat: 23g; Total Carbs: 14g; Fiber: 5g; Net Carbs: 9g; Protein: 5g MACROS - Fat: 76%; Protein: 4%; Carbs: 20%

PROSCIUTTO-WRAPPED ASPARAGUS

PREP TIME: 5 MINUTES | COOK TIME: 10 MINUTES

AIP-Elimination Phase Compliant

SERVES 2

Asparagus is rich in folate, antioxidants, and vitamins E and C, which makes it a great vegetable for an anti-inflammatory diet. This recipe only has four ingredients, cooks quickly, and is the perfect complement to beef, chicken, or seafood.

12 asparagus spears, woody ends removed

4 slices prosciutto

2 tablespoons avocado oil

½ teaspoon salt

1. Preheat the oven to 400°F. Line a baking sheet with parchment paper.

2. Divide the asparagus spears into four equal parts. Securely wrap each of the bundles with a slice of prosciutto around the middle.

3. Drizzle the avocado oil over top of the bundles and sprinkle with salt.

4. Bake for 10 minutes.

Tip: Hold each asparagus spear and bend the stalk until it snaps. This will ensure that you end up with only the tender top part of each spear and the woody ends are removed.

Per Serving Calories: 270; Total Fat: 23g; Total Carbs: 4g; Fiber: 2g; Net Carbs:2g; Protein: 14g MACROS – Fat: 75%; Protein: 20%; Carbs: 5%

BROCCOLI AND SHALLOTS

PREP TIME: 5 MINUTES | COOK TIME: 15 MINUTES

AIP-Elimination Phase Compliant

SERVES 2

Broccoli is full of vitamins C and K, calcium, and other nutrients like magnesium, zinc, and phosphorous, making it perfect for an anti-inflammatory diet. Plus it tastes especially delicious when it is roasted in the oven! This side dish takes only 20 minutes to make and is full of vibrant flavors. It will soon be a weeknight staple.

3 cups broccoli, chopped into florets

½ large shallot, peeled and thinly sliced

2 cloves garlic, minced

2 tablespoons avocado oil

1 teaspoon lemon juice

¼ teaspoon salt

1. Preheat the oven to 425°F. Line a baking sheet with parchment paper.

2. Place the broccoli florets, shallots, and garlic cloves onto the baking sheet.

3. Pour the avocado oil over the broccoli, shallots, and garlic and toss to coat completely.

4. Arrange the vegetables in a single layer and roast for 20 minutes or until the broccoli is tender.

5. Top with the lemon juice and sprinkle with salt.

Swap: You can substitute the avocado oil for ghee or grass-fed butter if they have been successfully reintroduced.

Per Serving Calories: 175; Total Fat: 15g; Total Carbs: 10g; Fiber: 4g; Net Carbs: 6g; Protein: 4g MACROS · Fat: 73%; Protein: 6%; Carbs: 21%

SAUTÉED SUPER GREENS

PREP TIME: 5 MINUTES | COOK TIME: 10 MINUTES

AIP-Elimination Phase Compliant

SERVES 2

When it comes to nutrients, leafy greens are powerhouses. They are chock-full of vitamins A, C, and K, plus potassium and fiber. Mix and match your favorite greens in this recipe.

2 tablespoons avocado oil

4 cloves garlic, minced

4 cups greens (spinach, kale, chard, or collards), coarsely chopped

1 teaspoon apple cider vinegar

1 teaspoon salt

1. In a large skillet, heat the oil over medium heat.

2. Add the garlic into the skillet and sauté for 5 minutes.

3. Add the greens and continue to sauté for 10 minutes or until tender.

4. Stir in the vinegar and salt.

Tip: We are garlic obsessed at Clean Keto Lifestyle and we love to cook with a lot of garlic! If you aren't a big garlic fan, feel free to use less or omit altogether.

Swap: You can substitute the avocado oil for ghee or grass-fed butter if these have been successfully reintroduced.

Per Serving Calories: 158; Total Fat: 14g; Total Carbs: 5g; Fiber: 1g; Net Carbs: 4g; Protein: 3g MACROS - Fat: 80%; Protein: 7%; Carbs: 13%

CUCUMBER HERB SALAD

PREP TIME: 5 MINUTES

AIP-Elimination Phase Compliant

SERVES 2

This recipe is inspired by the lively flavors of Greece and is light and refreshing. Make this salad the night before to allow the flavors to marry. You can also turn this dish into a complete meal by topping it with a roasted chicken thigh, baked salmon fillet, or mixing in some canned tuna.

1 cucumber, halved
   lengthwise, seeded, and
   diced into ½-inch pieces
½ cup red onion,
   thinly sliced
½ cup Greek Vinaigrette
   (page 176)

1. In a large bowl, mix the cucumbers and onion.
2. Pour the Greek Vinaigrette into the bowl and toss to combine.

Swap: Feel free to add in some goat cheese, feta, or tomatoes if these have been successfully reintroduced.

Per Serving Calories: 324; Total Fat: 32g; Total Carbs: 8g; Fiber: 1g; Net Carbs: 7g; Protein: 1g MACROS - Fat: 89%; Protein: 1%; Carbs: 10%

CRISPED BRUSSELS SPROUTS
WITH SRIRACHA AIOLI

PREP TIME: 10 MINUTES | COOK TIME: 25 MINUTES

AIP-Reintroduction Phase: Non-AIP Spices (black pepper),
Eggs & Egg-Based Sauces (mayo), Nightshades (sriracha)

SERVES 8

Oven-roasting Brussels sprouts brings out a lovely nutty flavor and the outsides take on a nice crispy texture. We paired these roasted Brussels sprouts with a spicy Sriracha Aioli that makes this side dish irresistible.

FOR THE BRUSSELS SPROUTS

2 pounds Brussels sprouts, small and medium ones cut in half and large ones cut in quarters

¼ cup avocado oil

1 teaspoon salt

¼ teaspoon black pepper

¼ cup plain pork rinds, crushed (optional)

TO MAKE THE BRUSSELS SPROUTS

1. Preheat the oven to 400°F. Line a baking sheet with parchment paper.

2. Spread out the Brussels sprouts in a single layer on the baking sheet.

3. Fully coat the Brussels sprouts with the avocado oil, salt, and pepper.

4. Bake for 25 minutes or until they turn dark and crisped on the outsides.

FOR THE SRIRACHA AIOLI

1 tablespoon sriracha sauce

¼ cup avocado-oil based
   mayonnaise (like Primal
   Kitchen brand)

⅛ teaspoon garlic powder

2 teaspoons lemon juice

TO MAKE THE SIRIRACHA AIOLI

5. In a small bowl, make the Sriracha Aioli by mixing together the sriracha, mayonnaise, garlic powder, and lemon juice.

6. When the Brussels sprouts are done cooking, drizzle with aioli, and then top with the crushed pork rinds (if using).

Tips: Opt for an organic sriracha sauce that doesn't include any additives. Also, the pork rinds add a nice crunch to this dish, but are optional.

Per Serving Calories: 145; Total Fat: 10g; Total Carbs: 11g; Fiber: 5g; Net Carbs: 6g; Protein: 4g MACROS - Fat: 62%; Protein: 8%; Carbs: 30%

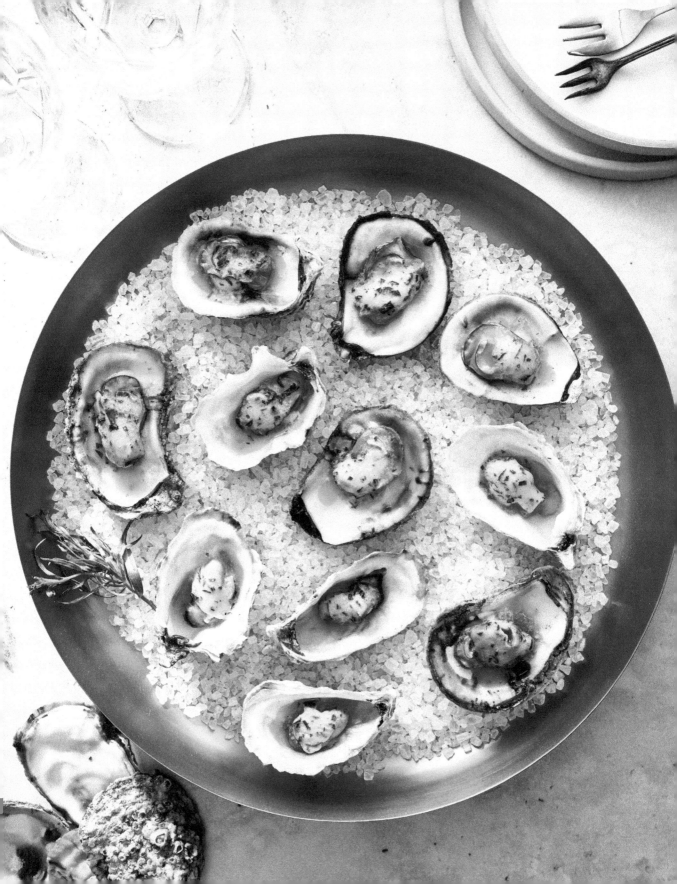

Chapter 5

SNACKS AND APPETIZERS

CRISPY KALE

PREP TIME: 5 MINUTES | COOK TIME: 15 MINUTES

AIP-Elimination Phase Compliant

SERVES 8

Crispy Kale is the perfect snack when you need a salty, crunchy bite. These kale chips are perfect to have on hand throughout the week.

2½ pounds curly kale

¼ cup avocado oil

1 teaspoon salt

½ teaspoon garlic powder

1. Preheat the oven to 350°F. Line a baking sheet with parchment paper.
2. Lay each kale leaf on a cutting board and cut out the stem with a knife. Tear the larger leaves in half.
3. In a large bowl, toss the kale with the avocado oil, salt, and garlic powder.
4. Spread the kale out in a single layer on the baking sheet. Bake for 15 minutes or until crisped.

Tip: Store in a sealed container at room temperature for up to 7 days.

Per Serving Calories: 148; Total Fat: 9g; Total Carbs: 14g; Fiber: 4g; Net Carbs: 10g; Protein: 5g MACROS · Fat: 54%; Protein: 11%; Carbs: 35%

GARLIC ROSEMARY ZUCCHINI CHIPS

PREP TIME: 10 MINUTES | COOK TIME: 2 HOURS

AIP-Elimination Phase Compliant

SERVES 8

Crispy and seasoned to perfection, zucchini chips make a great low-carb alternative to potato chips! Eat these chips plain or pair them with our Cucumber Tzatziki (page 181) or our Sweet Horseradish Cream (page 180).

4 zucchinis

2 tablespoons avocado oil

½ teaspoon garlic powder

½ teaspoon salt

1 teaspoon finely
   chopped rosemary

1. Using a knife or mandoline, thinly slice the zucchinis. A mandoline will give you thin and uniform chips.

2. Lay the slices on paper towels without overlapping. Place another layer of paper towels on top. Lay a baking sheet on top of the paper towels to press out the moisture. Let sit for 15 minutes.

3. Preheat the oven to 235°F. Line the same baking sheet with parchment paper.

4. Brush half the avocado oil on the parchment paper.

5. Once the moisture has been removed from the zucchini slices, arrange the slices on the lined baking sheet in a single layer and brush the remaining avocado oil on top of the slices.

6. In a small bowl, mix together the garlic powder, salt, and rosemary. Sprinkle on top of the zucchini slices.

7. Bake for 1½ hours to 2 hours or until crisped.

Tips: Try to find the fattest zucchini you can, as the chips will shrink considerably while baking. You can store these chips at room temperature in a sealed container for up to 3 days.

Per Serving Calories: 47; Total Fat: 4g; Total Carbs: 2g; Fiber: 1g; Net Carbs: 1g; Protein: 1g MACROS - Fat: 76%; Protein: 7%; Carbs: 17%

BLACKBERRY COCONUT CUPS

PREP TIME: 5 MINUTES, 30 MINUTES TO FREEZE

AIP-Elimination Phase Compliant

MAKES 12 COCONUT CUPS

This is our Autoimmune Keto version of a fat bomb. They are the perfect bite-sized treat and pack a major healthy fat punch! Blackberries have the lowest net carb count of all the types of berries and are packed with essential nutrients and antioxidants. They contain a high level of vitamins C, K, and A, as well as anthocyanins (which are antioxidants that fight against free radicals in the body).

1 cup coconut butter (also called manna)

1 cup coconut oil

½ cup blackberries (fresh or frozen)

1 teaspoon ground cinnamon

½ teaspoon salt

1. Place a cupcake liner in each well of a 12-cup muffin tin.

2. Put coconut butter, coconut oil, blackberries, cinnamon, and salt into a food processor or blender. Process until smooth and thick.

3. Pour the batter evenly into the cupcake liners and freeze for 30 minutes before serving.

4. Store the Blackberry Coconut Cups in a sealed container in the freezer for up to 7 days.

Swap: Feel free to swap out the blackberries for ½ cup of raspberries, strawberries, or blueberries.

Per Serving Calories: 266; Total Fat: 29g; Total Carbs: 5g; Fiber: 3g; Net Carbs: 2g; Protein: 1g MACROS · Fat: 92%; Protein: 2%; Carbs: 6%

STICKY WINGS

PREP TIME: 5 MINUTES | COOK TIME: 25 MINUTES

AIP-Elimination Phase Compliant

SERVES 8

These crowd-pleasing wings are sweet, sticky, and absolutely delicious. No one would ever guess that they are completely keto and AIP-compliant! With a very short prep and cook time, these wings are a fast and easy appetizer option.

40 chicken wings

1 tablespoon salt

1 tablespoon garlic powder

¼ cup coconut aminos

2 tablespoons fish sauce (like Red Boat brand)

4 teaspoons grated ginger root

2 teaspoons raw honey

1 tablespoon fresh cilantro, chopped, for garnish (optional)

1. Preheat the oven to 425°F. Line a baking sheet with parchment paper.

2. Pat the wings dry with a paper towel.

3. Place the wings on the baking sheet and toss with the salt and garlic powder.

4. Bake for 20 to 25 minutes or until the internal temperature reaches 160°F.

5. While the wings are baking, prepare the sauce by mixing together the coconut aminos, fish sauce, ginger, and honey in a small bowl.

6. When the wings have reached 160°F, remove them from the oven and brush them with the sauce.

7. Place the wings back in the oven and bake for another 3 to 5 minutes or until the internal temperature reaches about 170°F.

8. Garnish with cilantro (if using) and serve.

Tip: Using a meat thermometer is a foolproof way to make sure your wings come out perfect every time.

Per Serving Calories: 549; Total Fat: 39g; Total Carbs: 1g; Fiber: 0g; Net Carbs: 1g; Protein: 45g MACROS - Fat: 64%; Protein: 35%; Carbs: 1%

GINGER CHICKEN MEATBALLS

PREP TIME: 5 MINUTES | COOK TIME: 15 MINUTES

AIP-Elimination Phase Compliant

SERVES 4

These meatballs are the perfect appetizer to serve at your next dinner party or game day get-together. They're fast, easy to make, and the recipe can be doubled or tripled to serve more people. They're a total crowd-pleaser!

FOR THE MEATBALLS

1 pound ground chicken

3 teaspoons grated ginger root

2 cloves garlic, minced

2 scallions, chopped

1 tablespoon coconut aminos

1 teaspoon fish sauce (like Red Boat brand)

1 tablespoon fresh cilantro, chopped

½ teaspoon salt

FOR THE SAUCE

2 tablespoons balsamic vinegar

2 tablespoons coconut aminos

1. Preheat the oven to 375°F. Line a baking sheet with parchment paper.

2. In a medium bowl, mix together the chicken, ginger, garlic, scallions, coconut aminos, fish sauce, cilantro, and salt until fully combined.

3. Form into 1½-inch balls, and place them on the baking sheet.

4. Bake for 15 minutes or until the internal temperature reaches 165°F.

5. In a small saucepan, heat the balsamic vinegar and coconut aminos over medium heat until bubbling. Reduce the heat to low and let it simmer for 5 minutes.

6. Drizzle the sauce over the cooked meatballs and garnish with cilantro.

Tip: For perfectly cooked chicken meatballs, we highly suggest using a meat thermometer to monitor the temperature and ensure that your meatballs stay tender and moist.

Per Serving Calories: 172; Total Fat: 9g; Total Carbs: 3g; Fiber: 0g; Net Carbs: 3g; Protein: 20g MACROS - Fat: 48%; Protein: 46%; Carbs: 6%

SPICED PECANS

PREP TIME: 5 MINUTES | COOK TIME: 15 MINUTES

AIP-Reintroduction Phase: Nightshades (paprika, cayenne pepper),
Non-AIP Spices (cumin), Nuts (pecans), Eggs & Egg-Based Sauces

SERVES 12

These Spiced Pecans are the perfect mix of sweet and salty, making them a great snack to keep on hand. Pecans are rich in vitamins A, B, and E, folic acid, calcium, potassium, and zinc, plus they are full of healthy fats and low in net carbs, which makes them the perfect keto nut.

3 cups pecan halves

1 egg white, beaten

1 tablespoon
   smoked paprika

2 teaspoons coconut sugar

1½ teaspoons
   ground cinnamon

1 teaspoon cayenne pepper

1 teaspoon salt

1 teaspoon ground cumin

¼ teaspoon garlic powder

1. Preheat the oven to 300°F. Line a baking sheet with parchment paper.

2. In a large bowl, mix together the pecans and egg whites.

3. In a small bowl, mix together the paprika, coconut sugar, cinnamon, cayenne, salt, cumin, and garlic powder.

4. Pour the spice mixture onto the pecans and toss gently to coat.

5. Spread the pecans in a single layer on the baking sheet and bake for 15 minutes.

6. Let them cool completely before eating.

Tip: Check on the pecans often while they are baking to ensure they don't burn.

Swap: To lower the carb content, you can swap out the coconut sugar for 2 teaspoons of erythritol if it has been successfully reintroduced.

Per Serving Calories: 198; Total Fat: 20g; Total Carbs: 4g; Fiber: 3g; Net Carbs: 1g; Protein: 5g MACROS · Fat: 83%; Protein: 9%; Carbs: 8%

OYSTERS WITH TARRAGON TABASCO

PREP TIME: 5 MINUTES, PLUS 1 HOUR TO CHILL | COOK TIME: 10 MINUTES

AIP-Reintroduction Phase: Dairy (ghee & butter), Nightshades (Tabasco sauce)

SERVES 6 TO 8

Oysters are rich in zinc, omega-3 fatty acids, potassium, magnesium, vitamins A, E, and C, selenium, iron, and vitamin B_{12}. Don't be intimidated to cook these, as the grilling process will pop the shells open for you. If an outdoor grill isn't available, put them in a roasting pan filled with ⅓-inch water and bake in the oven at 475°F for 7 to 10 minutes.

8 tablespoons ghee or grass-fed butter

1 tablespoon Tabasco sauce

2 tablespoons chopped tarragon

⅛ teaspoon garlic powder

⅛ teaspoon onion powder

¼ teaspoon salt

36 fresh raw oysters in their shells

1. In a small bowl, mix together the ghee, Tabasco, tarragon, garlic powder, onion powder, and salt. Put the mixture in plastic wrap and roll it into a log. Refrigerate for 1 hour.

2. Heat your grill to high.

3. Place the oysters on the grill and cook for 5 to 10 minutes, or until the oysters pop open.

4. Carefully remove the top shell, leaving the oyster in the bottom shell.

5. Put a portion of the refrigerated ghee mixture on each oyster and place the oyster back on the grill to melt the ghee. Serve immediately.

Tips: Discard any opened oysters before cooking and any unopened oysters after cooking. You will usually get several that are not safe to eat, so always buy more oysters than you think you'll need. Use a grill mitt and tongs to handle the hot shells. Also, when prying open the oysters, try to keep the oyster liquor inside the shell—it is packed with a lovely flavor.

Per Serving Calories: 181; Total Fat: 17g; Total Carbs: 2g; Fiber: 0g; Net Carbs: 2g; Protein: 5g MACROS - Fat: 84%; Protein: 11%; Carbs: 5%

CEVICHE BAY SCALLOPS WITH ROASTED RED PEPPER AIOLI

PREP TIME: 5 MINUTES, PLUS 2 HOURS TO CHILL

AIP-Reintroduction Phase: Eggs & Egg-Based Sauces (mayo), Nightshades (tomatoes and red peppers), Non-AIP spices (black pepper)

SERVES 8

Bay scallops are the star of this elegant dish! Cooked with the acidity from the lemon juice, these scallops are perfectly complemented with a delicious Roasted Red Pepper Aioli. Serve as an appetizer or a tapas plate.

1 pound bay scallops

Juice from 1 lemon

2 tablespoons capers

¼ cup diced tomatoes

2 teaspoons fresh oregano, chopped

¼ cup watercress

4 tablespoons Roasted Red Pepper Aioli, divided

FOR THE ROASTED RED PEPPER AIOLI

2 whole roasted red peppers

⅔ cup fresh basil

Juice from ½ lemon

2 cloves garlic, minced

1½ cups avocado-oil based mayonnaise (like Primal Kitchen brand)

½ teaspoon salt

¼ teaspoon black pepper

1. In a medium bowl, toss the scallops and lemon juice.
2. Cover and refrigerate for 2 hours.
3. Remove the scallops from the refrigerator and strain the juice.
4. Add the capers, tomatoes, oregano, watercress, and 1 tablespoon of the Roasted Red Pepper Aioli to the scallops and toss gently.
5. Plate the dish by spreading the remaining 3 tablespoons of the Roasted Red Pepper Aioli on the bottom of a plate and topping it with the scallop mixture.

FOR THE ROASTED RED PEPPER AIOLI

Put the red peppers, basil, lemon juice, garlic, mayonnaise, salt, and pepper in a food processor or blender; process until smooth.

Tip: You can also serve this dish tapas-style by serving on eight individual plates to eight people.

Per Serving Calories: 389; Total Fat: 37g; Total Carbs: 4g; Fiber: 1g; Net Carbs: 3g; Protein: 10g MACROS - Fat: 85%; Protein: 10%; Carbs: 5%

PESTO SWIRL ROLLS

PREP TIME: 30 MINUTES, PLUS 2 HOURS TO RISE | COOK TIME: 25 MINUTES

AIP-Reintroduction Phase: Dairy (ghee), Eggs &
Egg-Based Sauces, Nuts (almond milk)

MAKES 10 ROLLS

These low-carb rolls have a beautiful and fluffy texture and a pop of flavor with the pesto. If you have successfully reintroduced dairy, add a sprinkle of cheddar cheese to make these even tastier. Make sure to plan ahead when making these since it takes 2 full hours for the dough to rise before baking.

¾ cup almond milk, warmed

2 teaspoons active
   dry yeast

2 teaspoons raw honey

2 eggs, plus 1 egg white

2 tablespoons ghee, melted

3 cups almond flour

¼ cup coconut flour

2 teaspoons xanthan gum

½ teaspoon salt

¼ cup Basil Pesto (see
   recipe on page 174)

1 teaspoon fresh thyme,
   chopped, for garnish

1. In a small bowl, mix the almond milk, yeast, and honey. Let sit for 10 minutes. The mixture should look foamy.

2. In a large bowl, beat the eggs, egg white, and ghee together with an electric or stand mixer until fluffy.

3. In another large bowl, mix the almond flour, coconut flour, xanthan gum, and salt together.

4. Pour the yeast mixture into the egg mixture and beat.

5. Slowly stir in the flour mixture until fully combined and a dough forms.

6. Cover the bowl with a towel and let the dough sit in a draft-free area for one hour.

7. After one hour, roll out the dough into a 16-by-10-inch rectangle between two layers of parchment paper.

8. Spread the pesto on top of the dough.

9. Roll the dough up tightly lengthwise into a log shape.

10. Cut the dough into 10 slices and place each slice in a 9-by-13-inch casserole dish.

11. Cover with a towel and let it rise again for another hour.

12. Bake the rolls at 350°F for 20 to 25 minutes or until golden brown.

13. Garnish with fresh thyme.

Tip: To get the most rise out of your rolls, try turning your oven on to the "warm" setting. Set your bowl of dough on top of the oven (not inside the oven) and let the warm air rise to help your rolls fluff.

Per Serving (1 roll) Calories: 144; Total Fat: 11g; Total Carbs: 6g; Fiber: 3g; Net Carbs: 3g; Protein: 5g MACROS - Fat: 67%; Protein: 13%; Carbs: 20%

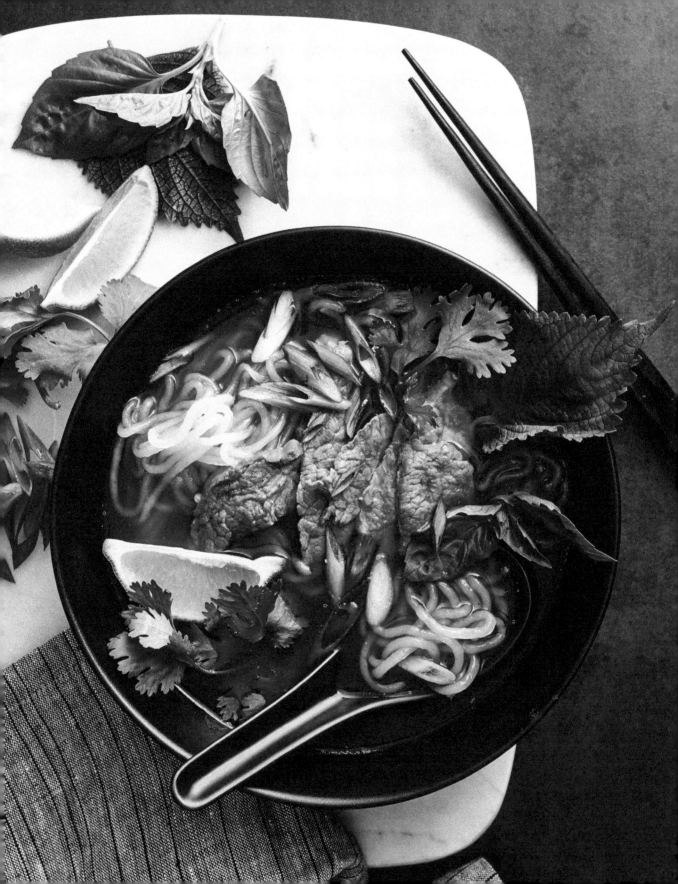

Chapter 6

SOUPS AND SALADS

HEALING CHICKEN SOUP

PREP TIME: 5 MINUTES | COOK TIME: 35 MINUTES

AIP-Elimination Phase Compliant

SERVES 4

This is not your store-bought chicken soup! We upgraded ordinary chicken soup with fresh veggies, healing bone broth, and flavorful herbs. It is a hearty, warming, go-to favorite for the AIP-Elimination Phase.

4 tablespoons avocado oil

¼ cup carrots, chopped into ½-inch pieces

½ cup celery, chopped into ½-inch pieces

½ cup yellow onion, diced

2 cloves garlic, minced

6 cups Chicken Bone Broth (store-bought or homemade, page 166)

1½ tablespoons fresh parsley, chopped

1 bay leaf

1 teaspoon salt

8 skinless, boneless chicken thighs

1 (14 ounce) can full-fat coconut milk

1 tablespoon coconut flour

2 avocados, diced

1. In a large pot, heat the oil over medium heat. Add the carrot, celery, and onion, and sauté for about 4 minutes until soft.

2. Add the garlic and sauté for another minute.

3. Add the bone broth, parsley, bay leaf, salt, and chicken thighs to the pot.

4. Bring to a boil, then cover with a lid and reduce the heat to low and let it simmer for 10 to 15 minutes or until the chicken is cooked through.

5. Remove the chicken and allow it to cool for 5 minutes before shredding it using two forks.

6. In a small saucepan, combine the coconut milk and coconut flour over medium heat and cook for 5 minutes.

7. Whisk the coconut milk mixture into the soup.

8. Return the shredded chicken to the soup and stir to combine.

9. Top with the diced avocado just before serving.

Tip: This soup is a great way to use up any leftover vegetables and fresh herbs that have been sitting around, such as zucchini, leeks, rosemary, or thyme.

Per Serving Calories: 626; Total Fat: 50g; Total Carbs: 16g; Fiber: 8g; Net Carbs: 8g; Protein: 28g MACROS - Fat: 73%; Protein: 17%; Carbs: 10%

CAULIFLOWER AND BACON SOUP

PREP TIME: 5 MINUTES | COOK TIME: 35 MINUTES

AIP-Elimination Phase Compliant

SERVES 3

This Cauliflower and Bacon Soup packs a flavor punch and couldn't be easier to make. The bacon provides incredible flavor and the cauliflower adds a rich, silky creaminess.

6 slices bacon (nitrate-free, no sugar added), cut into ½-inch pieces

1 yellow onion, chopped

3 cloves garlic, minced

6 cups Chicken Bone Broth (store-bought or homemade, page 166)

1 cup full-fat coconut milk

1 head (about 4 cups) cauliflower, chopped into florets

1 teaspoon salt

1. In a large skillet, cook the bacon over medium heat for 10 to 12 minutes or until crisped. Transfer the bacon to a paper towel-lined plate. Reserve the bacon fat.

2. Pour the bacon fat in a large pot over medium heat.

3. Add the onion and garlic to the pot and sauté, stirring constantly until onion is softened, about 5 minutes.

4. Add the bone broth, coconut milk, cauliflower, and salt to the pot.

5. Cover and cook for 30 minutes or until the cauliflower is completely tender.

6. Using an immersion blender, blend the soup until completely smooth.

7. Garnish with the cooked bacon pieces.

Tip: If the soup is too thick, whisk in additional bone broth until you've reached the desired consistency. If you don't have an immersion blender, transfer the soup to a blender in batches and purée. Check the ingredients on the bacon package and ensure any added spices are AIP-friendly.

Per Serving Calories: 382; Total Fat: 26g; Total Carbs: 15g; Fiber: 5g; Net Carbs: 10g; Protein: 22g MACROS - Fat: 62%; Protein: 24%; Carbs: 14%

TOM KHA GAI

PREP TIME: 5 MINUTES | COOK TIME: 40 MINUTES

AIP-Elimination Phase Compliant

SERVES 2

This coconut milk-based soup is aromatic and flavorful thanks to all the classic Thai ingredients used in the recipe like lemongrass, ginger, and lime. You can find fresh lemongrass in the produce section of almost every grocery store. If you can't find it fresh, look for lemongrass paste in a tube.

1 stalk fresh lemongrass, outer layers removed

1-inch piece ginger, peeled

4 cups Chicken Bone Broth (store-bought or homemade, page 166)

2 tablespoons lime juice

½ tablespoon lime zest

4 skinless, boneless chicken thighs, cut into 1-inch pieces

1 cup white button mushrooms, cut into pieces

1 cup full-fat coconut milk

1 tablespoon fish sauce (like Red Boat brand)

1 teaspoon raw honey

2 tablespoons fresh cilantro, chopped (optional)

1 lime, cut into 6 wedges

1. With the back of a knife, lightly smash the lemongrass and ginger.

2. Cut the lemongrass into separate 4-inch pieces.

3. In a large pot, bring the lemongrass, ginger, bone broth, lime juice, and lime zest to a boil, then reduce the heat to low and let it simmer for 10 minutes.

4. Use a slotted spoon to remove the lemongrass and ginger pieces from the soup, as well as scrape off any other particulate that floats to the top.

5. Add the chicken to the broth and bring to a boil once again.

6. Reduce the heat to low and add in the mushrooms.

7. Cook for 25 minutes then stir in the coconut milk, fish sauce, honey, and cilantro (if using).

8. Serve with lime wedges.

Tip: Bruising the lemongrass and ginger help them release their oils and flavors, so don't skip this first step!

Per Serving Calories: 556; Total Fat: 36g; Total Carbs: 9g; Fiber: 3g; Net Carbs: 6g; Protein: 49g MACROS - Fat: 60%; Protein: 35%; Carbs: 5%

BEEF PHO

AIP-Elimination Phase Compliant

SERVES 6

There are few things better than the warm aroma of ginger, cinnamon, and garlic simmering on the stovetop. Made with bone broth, which is full of collagen and gut-healing properties, our nourishing version of Beef Pho is wonderfully filling and perfect for an anti-inflammatory diet.

10 cups Beef Bone Broth (store-bought or homemade, page 168)

1 (6-inch) piece of ginger, peeled and cut in half lengthwise

1 cinnamon stick

4 cloves garlic

¼ cup fish sauce (like Red Boat brand)

2 teaspoons raw honey

1 teaspoon salt

1 pound flank steak, finely sliced against the grain

1 (7 ounce) package shirataki noodles, prepared according to the package instructions

¼ cup whole Thai basil leaves, torn into pieces

¼ cup fresh cilantro, chopped

2 scallions, chopped

1 lime, cut into 6 wedges

1. In a large pot, combine the bone broth, ginger, cinnamon, garlic, fish sauce, honey, and salt.

2. Bring the broth to a boil, then cover with a lid and reduce the heat to low, and let it simmer for at least 30 minutes.

3. Use a slotted spoon to remove the ginger pieces, cinnamon sticks, and garlic cloves from the soup, as well as scrape off any other particulate that floats to the top.

4. Divide the steak, shirataki noodles, basil, cilantro, and scallions into 6 bowls and pour the hot broth into each one. The steak and noodles will cook in the broth.

5. Serve with lime wedges.

Tip: Shirataki noodles can be found in the refrigerated section of the grocery store and are the perfect replacement for pasta. Plus, they contain resistant starch, which fuels your good gut bacteria. Our favorite brand is Miracle Noodles.

Swap: The Thai basil leaves can be substituted with regular basil.

Per Serving Calories: 190; Total Fat: 7g; Total Carbs: 7g; Fiber: 1g; Net Carbs: 6g; Protein: 23g MACROS - Fat: 34%; Protein: 51%; Carbs: 15%

ARTICHOKE AND HEARTS OF PALM SALAD

PREP TIME: 10 MINUTES | COOK TIME: 30 MINUTES

AIP-Elimination Phase Compliant

SERVES 2

The artichokes, hearts of palm, and avocados pump up the anti-inflammatory benefits of this delicious salad. It is the perfect dish to make when you are in the mood for something clean and healthy, but also satisfying. Make the chicken ahead of time so you can assemble the salad in just a few minutes.

4 skin-on chicken thighs

1 tablespoon avocado oil

½ teaspoon salt

8 cups mixed greens

½ (14 ounce) can of artichokes, drained and cut in quarters

½ (14 ounce) can sliced hearts of palm, drained

2 avocados, sliced

½ cup Autoimmune Keto House Dressing (page 177)

1. Preheat the oven to 400°F. Line a baking sheet with parchment paper.

2. Coat the chicken thighs with avocado oil and season with salt.

3. Place the chicken on the baking sheet and roast in the oven for 20 to 30 minutes or until the juices run clear. Let cool slightly and dice into 1-inch pieces.

4. Assemble the salad by placing the greens, artichokes, hearts of palm, chicken, and avocado in a large bowl.

5. Pour the dressing over the salad and toss to incorporate.

Tip: Since you use only ½ can of both the artichokes and hearts of palm in this recipe, make a marinade by combining the juice of 1 lemon, 2 tablespoons of extra-virgin olive oil, 2 teaspoons dried oregano, 1 teaspoon garlic powder, 1 teaspoon thyme, and ½ teaspoon salt. Put the artichokes and hearts of palm in a glass jar, pour over the marinade, seal the jar, and store in the refrigerator for up to 7 days.

Per Serving Calories: 1129; Total Fat: 93g; Total Carbs: 30g; Fiber: 16g; Net Carbs: 7g; Protein: 43g MACROS - Fat: 74%; Protein: 15%; Carbs: 11%

CUCUMBER AND BEEF MINT SALAD

PREP TIME: 10 MINUTES | COOK TIME: 10 MINUTES

AIP-Elimination Phase Compliant

SERVES 2

This elegant salad has a lovely contrast of flavors and an upscale feel. It is versatile enough to make as a quick lunch, or you can easily increase the recipe to serve for a fancy dinner party.

12-ounce skirt steak

1 cucumber, sliced into thin ribbons (about 2 cups)

⅔ cups fresh mint leaves, whole

1 avocado, sliced

FOR THE DRESSING

2 cloves garlic, minced

3 tablespoons lime juice

1 tablespoon fish sauce (like Red Boat brand)

1 tablespoon fresh cilantro, chopped

1 teaspoon pure maple syrup

½ teaspoon salt

¼ cup extra-virgin olive oil

1 tablespoon shallots, diced

1. Heat your grill or grill pan to high heat. Cook the steak on the grill for about 10 minutes or until the internal temperature reaches 120 to 125°F, flipping halfway through.

2. Transfer the steak to a plate, and let it rest for 10 minutes before slicing it against the grain. The internal temperature should rise to 130 to 135°F.

3. While the steak is resting, prepare the dressing by mixing the garlic, lime juice, fish sauce, cilantro, maple syrup, and salt in a bowl. Slowly whisk in the olive oil until well combined.

4. Next, add in the shallots and mix well.

5. In a salad bowl, mix together the cucumber ribbons and mint leaves.

6. Assemble the salad by plating the cucumber and mint first, followed by the steak, then topping with the dressing and sliced avocado.

Swaps: You can top this salad with chopped almonds if you have successfully reintroduced nuts. Also, if you have successfully reintroduced them, we recommend adding 2 small red chilies that are seeded and thinly sliced to the dressing to add a spicy kick.

Per Serving Calories: 675; Total Fat: 51g; Total Carbs: 14g; Fiber: 6g; Net Carbs: 8g; Protein: 40g MACROS - Fat: 69%; Protein: 24%; Carbs: 7%

SUBMARINE DELUXE SALAD

PREP TIME: 10 MINUTES

AIP-Reintroduction Phase: Nightshades (tomatoes, banana peppers),
Non-AIP spices (salami spices)

SERVES 6

Who needs bread when you can take all the best parts of a traditional submarine sandwich and make it into a salad? This Submarine Deluxe Salad is full of crisp vegetables and tossed with a tangy, tasty Greek Vinaigrette dressing. The result is pure perfection!

6 cups romaine
  lettuce, chopped
12 ounces nitrate-free
  salami, chopped
1 cup cherry
  tomatoes, halved
½ cup cucumber, sliced
½ cup black olives
½ cup banana
  peppers, sliced
½ cup Greek Vinaigrette
  (page 176)

1. Assemble the salad by placing the lettuce, salami, tomatoes, cucumber, olives, and banana peppers in a large bowl.

2. Pour the Greek Vinaigrette over the salad and toss to combine.

Swaps: Feel free to swap out the salami for an equal amount of prosciutto, pepperoni, capicola, or a combination of all of them.

Per Serving Calories: 295; Total Fat: 27g; Total Carbs: 5g; Fiber: 2g; Net Carbs: 3g; Protein: 8g MACROS - Fat: 82%; Protein: 11%; Carbs: 7%

PISTACHIO POMEGRANATE SALAD

PREP TIME: 10 MINUTES | COOK TIME: 10 MINUTES

AIP-Reintroduction Phase: Dairy (cheese), Non-AIP Spices
(mustard, black pepper), Nuts (pistachios)

SERVES 4

Pistachios and pomegranate seeds are the stars of this gorgeous salad. Feel free to
swap out the pistachios for other low-carb nuts such as macadamia nuts, pecans,
and walnuts. This salad looks incredibly festive, making it perfect to serve around
the holidays.

FOR THE SALAD

1 tablespoon avocado oil

2 shallots, thinly sliced

6 cups baby spinach

3 tablespoons
pomegranate seeds

3 tablespoons
pistachios, shelled

2 ounces goat cheese
or Manchego
cheese (optional)

FOR THE DRESSING

1 tablespoon Dijon mustard

½ teaspoon salt

¼ teaspoon black pepper

1 clove garlic, minced

¼ cup balsamic vinegar

¾ cup extra-virgin olive oil

1. In a small skillet, heat the avocado oil over
    medium heat and add in the shallots. Sauté for
    5 minutes or until the shallots are soft, then
    remove from heat and let cool.

2. Make the dressing by combining the mustard,
    salt, pepper, garlic, and vinegar together in bowl.
    Slowly pour in the olive oil, whisking vigorously
    for 1 to 2 minutes.

3. Assemble the salad by placing the spinach, shal-
    lots, pomegranate seeds, pistachios, and cheese
    (if using) in a large bowl.

4. Pour desired amount of dressing over the salad
    and toss to combine.

Tip: Goat and sheep's milk cheese contain the A2 casein
protein, which is much less inflammatory than the A1 casein
protein found in cow's milk. One of the best ways to reintroduce dairy is to try goat and sheep's milk first and see how
your body reacts to it.

*Per Serving Calories: 460; Total Fat: 47g; Total Carbs: 9g; Fiber: 2g;
Net Carbs: 7g; Protein: 3g MACROS - Fat: 90%; Protein: 2%; Carbs: 8%*

BACON AND BERRY HARVEST SALAD

PREP TIME: 20 MINUTES

AIP-Reintroduction Phase: Dairy (goat cheese), Eggs & Egg-Based Sauces, Non-AIP Spices (mustard), Nuts (pecans)

SERVES 4

This recipe has lovely autumnal vibes courtesy of the warm flavors from the caramelized shallots, bacon, pecans, and eggs. We love how the dark color of the blackberries pops against the brown and earthy tones of the other ingredients.

FOR THE SALAD

6 cups mixed greens

8 slices bacon (nitrate-free, no sugar added), cooked and chopped

½ cup pecans, toasted and chopped

4 hard-boiled eggs, chopped

¾ cup blackberries

3 ounces crumbled goat cheese (optional)

FOR THE DRESSING

4 tablespoons spicy brown mustard

4 tablespoons balsamic vinegar

2 cloves garlic, minced

1 tablespoon fresh thyme

⅔ cup extra-virgin olive oil

1. Make the dressing by combining the mustard, vinegar, garlic, and thyme together in bowl. Slowly pour in the olive oil, whisking vigorously for 1 to 2 minutes.

2. Assemble the salad by placing the greens, followed by the cooked bacon, pecans, hard-boiled eggs, blackberries, and cheese (if using) in a large bowl.

3. Pour desired amount of dressing over the salad and toss to combine.

Tips: For perfectly cooked bacon, cook it on a baking sheet in the oven at 360°F for 20 to 25 minutes, flipping halfway through.

Per Serving Calories: 656; Total Fat: 63g; Total Carbs: 10g; Fiber: 4g; Net Carbs: 6g; Protein: 16g MACROS · Fat: 84%; Protein: 9%; Carbs: 7%

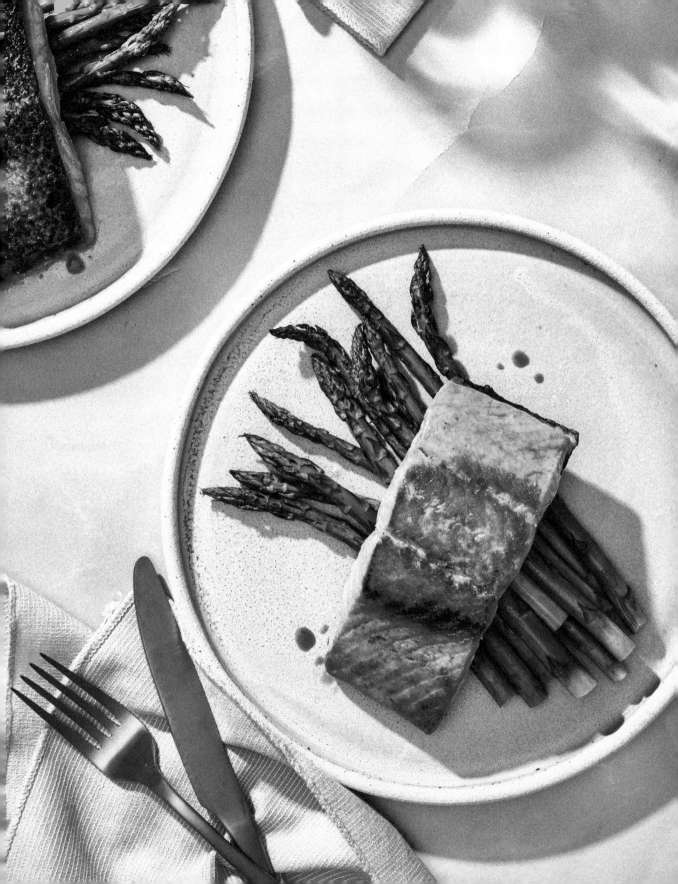

Chapter 7

POULTRY AND SEAFOOD

BACON-WRAPPED SCALLOPS WITH SWEET BALSAMIC SAUCE

PREP TIME: 5 MINUTES | COOK TIME: 25 MINUTES

AIP-Elimination Phase Compliant

SERVES 1

Scallops are rich in omega-3 fatty acids, vitamin B12, and antioxidants, which help to improve cardiovascular function and lower cholesterol levels. They also contain minerals like potassium and magnesium. But you'll love this easy dish because it tastes so decadent.

4 bacon slices (nitrate-free, no sugar added)

2 teaspoons balsamic vinegar, plus more for drizzling

2 teaspoons coconut aminos

6 ounces sea scallops, (approximately 4 medium-size)

1 tablespoon coconut oil

1. Preheat the oven to 360°F. Line a baking sheet with parchment paper.

2. Place the bacon on the baking sheet, cook for 10 minutes, then flip and cook for an additional 6 minutes. Transfer the bacon slices to a paper towel-lined plate. (You want the bacon to still be flexible enough to wrap around the scallops.)

3. In a small saucepan, heat the balsamic vinegar and coconut aminos on medium heat until bubbling. Reduce the heat and let simmer for 5 minutes.

4. Pat the scallops dry and wrap one slice of bacon around the circular edge of each scallop, folding the bacon down so that the scallop surface will still be touching the skillet.

5. Spear each scallop with a toothpick to secure the bacon around the scallops.

6. In a large skillet, heat the coconut oil over high heat.

7. Gently add the scallops flat-side down to the skillet, making sure you don't overcrowd your pan.

8. Cook for 2 to 3 minutes on each side.

9. Remove the scallops, put them on a plate, and drizzle the balsamic sauce over top.

Tip: Check the ingredients on the bacon package and ensure any added spices are AIP-friendly. Try to use thinly sliced bacon with a thin width for best results. Also, don't overcook your scallops or they will get tough and chewy.

Per Serving Calories: 447; Total Fat: 28g; Total Carbs: 6g; Fiber: 0g; Net Carbs: 6g; Protein: 40g MACROS - Fat: 57%; Protein: 37%; Carbs: 6%

TERIYAKI SHRIMP AND BROCCOLI

PREP TIME: 10 MINUTES | COOK TIME: 10 MINUTES

AIP-Elimination Phase Compliant

SERVES 1

Traditional teriyaki sauce contains sugar and soy, neither of which are AIP-Elimination Phase compliant. For a quick and easy dinner that is packed with flavor, make our upgraded Teriyaki Shrimp and Broccoli. Feel free to serve this over cauliflower rice or shirataki noodles.

FOR THE SAUCE

¼ cup Beef Bone Broth (store-bought or homemade, page 168)

1 clove garlic, minced

1 tablespoon coconut aminos

1 tablespoon balsamic vinegar

½ tablespoon fish sauce (like Red Boat brand)

½ tablespoon beef gelatin powder (like Great Lakes or Vital Proteins brand)

3 tablespoons filtered water, divided

1. Combine the bone broth, garlic, coconut aminos, balsamic vinegar, and fish sauce in a saucepan over medium heat.

2. Bring the sauce to a boil, then reduce it to a simmer.

3. Meanwhile, add the gelatin to a small bowl and bloom it by adding 1 tablespoon of lukewarm water to the gelatin, whisking vigorously, followed by 2 tablespoons of hot water, whisking vigorously again.

4. Slowly add the gelatin mixture to the sauce while continually whisking to mix it in thoroughly. Keep the sauce warmed over low heat and start on the shrimp.

FOR THE SHRIMP & BROCCOLI

2 tablespoons coconut oil

6 ounces shrimp, peeled and deveined

1 clove garlic, minced

½ teaspoon grated ginger root

2 cups broccoli, chopped into florets and steamed

TO MAKE THE SHRIMP

1. In a large skillet, heat the coconut oil over medium-high heat.

2. Add the shrimp, garlic, and ginger to the skillet and cook for about 4 minutes, flipping the shrimp halfway through.

3. When the shrimp are cooked through, turn the heat off and pour the sauce over the shrimp.

4. Serve the teriyaki shrimp over the steamed broccoli.

Swap: If you have successfully reintroduced nightshades, add some heat to your dish by using ½ teaspoon of red chili flakes or 1 teaspoon of sriracha sauce in the teriyaki sauce.

Per Serving Calories: 482; Total Fat: 31g; Total Carbs: 15g; Fiber: 6g; Net Carbs: 9g; Protein: 40g MACROS · Fat: 55%; Protein: 33%; Carbs: 12%

GARLIC LEMON COD WITH ASPARAGUS

PREP TIME: 5 MINUTES | COOK TIME: 15 MINUTES

AIP-Elimination Phase Compliant

SERVES 1

This is one of the first meals that we have our clients make on Autoimmune Keto. Preparing this simple and satisfying dish gives them the confidence they need to make eating like this a true lifestyle. Oh, and it is delicious, too!

2 tablespoons avocado oil, divided

2 cloves garlic, minced

6-ounce cod fillet

Juice from ½ lemon

1 tablespoon capers

¼ teaspoon salt

6 asparagus spears, woody ends removed

½ lemon, sliced thinly

1. Preheat the oven to 425°F. Line a baking sheet with parchment paper.

2. Combine 1 tablespoon of avocado oil and the garlic in a bowl.

3. Place the cod fillet on the baking sheet.

4. Rub the cod with the garlic and oil mixture until it is evenly coated.

5. Squeeze the lemon juice over the cod, top with the capers, and sprinkle with salt.

6. Arrange the asparagus around the cod in a single layer, drizzle the spears with the remaining avocado oil, and place the lemon slices over them.

7. Roast for 12 to 15 minutes, until the cod is cooked through.

Swaps: For more flavor, you can add ½ teaspoon of dried oregano. Feel free to use salmon, halibut, or sea bass in place of the cod.

Per Serving Calories: 415; Total Fat: 29g; Total Carbs: 6g; Fiber: 2g; Net Carbs: 4g; Protein: 33g MACROS - Fat: 62%; Protein: 32%; Carbs: 6%

CRISPY-SKIN SALMON

PREP TIME: 5 MINUTES | COOK TIME: 10 MINUTES

AIP-Elimination Phase Compliant

SERVES 1

Salmon skin contains the highest amounts of omega-3 fatty acids on the fish. Omega-3s are beneficial for every aspect of heart health and are essential for brain function and cell growth. Be sure to buy wild-caught salmon to reduce the risk of your fish being contaminated by pollutants.

6-ounce skin-on
   salmon fillet
¼ teaspoon salt
2 teaspoons
   coconut aminos

1. Pat the salmon dry, then sprinkle the skin side with salt (this will help absorb the excess moisture from the skin).

2. Heat a large skillet over medium heat.

3. Place the salmon skin-side down in the skillet. Cook for about 6 minutes.

4. Reduce the heat and pour the coconut aminos over the top of the salmon.

5. Flip the salmon carefully and cook for 1 to 2 more minutes until the internal temperature reaches 130°F for medium or 145°F for well done.

Tip: The side of asparagus in the Garlic Lemon Cod with Asparagus recipe (page 114) tastes great with this salmon dish as well.

Swap: For more flavor, you can mix in 2 teaspoons of grated ginger root to the coconut aminos.

Per Serving Calories: 239; Total Fat: 11g; Total Carbs: 2g; Fiber: 0g; Net Carbs: 2g; Protein: 33g MACROS · Fat: 40%; Protein: 59%; Carbs: 1%

PESTO HALIBUT IN PARCHMENT PAPER

PREP TIME: 5 MINUTES | COOK TIME: 20 MINUTES

AIP-Elimination Phase Compliant

1 SERVING

Baking the halibut in parchment paper preserves the tenderness of the fish. It also makes for quick cleanup, which is ideal on those busy weeknights. We paired the halibut with our AIP-friendly Basil Pesto to provide a burst of flavor to this dish.

6-ounce halibut fillet

1 sheet parchment
  paper, cut into a
  14-by-12-inch piece

2 tablespoons avocado oil

2 tablespoons Basil Pesto
  (page 174)

1. Preheat the oven to 375°F.

2. Place the halibut fillet on the sheet of parchment paper.

3. Brush the avocado oil onto the halibut and then spoon the Basil Pesto on top.

4. Close the parchment paper by folding in all four sides to completely enclose the fish.

5. Place the fish packet on a baking sheet and roast for 20 minutes until the halibut is opaque throughout.

6. Transfer the packet to a plate, open carefully, and serve.

Swap: Feel free to add ½ cup of halved cherry tomatoes to the packet if they have been successfully reintroduced.

Per Serving Calories: 547; Total Fat: 42g; Total Carbs: 3g; Fiber: 1g; Net Carbs: 2g; Protein: 35g MACROS - Fat: 70%; Protein: 27%; Carbs: 3%

CAJUN SHRIMP AND SAUSAGE KEBAB SALAD

PREP TIME: 5 MINUTES | COOK TIME: 20 MINUTES

AIP-Reintroduction Phase: Dairy (sour cream), Eggs & Egg-Based Sauces (mayo), Nightshades (bell peppers), Non-AIP spices (andouille sausage spices, Cajun seasoning)

SERVES 6

These simple kebabs are a great way to enjoy vegetables and protein together. This recipe makes a fast weeknight meal, and can also be easily increased to feed a large crowd.

1 pound large shrimp, peeled and deveined

2 teaspoons Cajun Seasoning, divided (page 184)

1 pound andouille sausage, cut into ½-inch slices

1½ bell peppers, cut into 1-inch pieces

1 medium white onion, cut into 1-inch pieces

¼ cup avocado-oil mayonnaise (like Primal Kitchen Brand)

¼ cup sour cream

12 cups mixed greens

1. Soak 12 wooden skewers in water for 15 minutes.
2. Heat your grill or grill pan to medium heat.
3. Season the shrimp with 1 teaspoon of Cajun seasoning.
4. Thread the sausage, shrimp, peppers, and onions evenly onto the wooden skewers, alternating one by one to create the kebabs.
5. Grill the kebabs for about 20 minutes, rotating them every 5 minutes.
6. In a medium bowl, mix the mayonnaise, sour cream, and remaining 1 teaspoon of Cajun Seasoning.
7. Divide the greens among 6 bowls and spoon the sauce on top of the greens.
8. Top each bowl with 3 skewers and serve.

Tip: If you don't have an outdoor grill or grill pan, you can bake these in the oven at 375°F for 20 to 25 minutes.

Per Serving Calories: 465; Total Fat: 37g; Total Carbs: 6g; Fiber: 2g; Net Carbs: 4g; Protein: 27g MACROS · Fat: 72%; Protein: 23%; Carbs: 5%

CRANBERRY TURKEY MEATLOAF

PREP TIME: 10 MINUTES | COOK TIME: 40 MINUTES

AIP-Elimination Phase Compliant

SERVES 6

It can be Thanksgiving any day of the week when making this dish! With notes of sage, thyme, and cranberries, this turkey meatloaf tastes amazing. The recipe makes 6 mini loaves, which can be stored in a sealed container in the refrigerator for up to 3 days if you have any left over.

2 tablespoons avocado oil

¼ cup yellow onion, diced

¼ cup celery, diced

2 cloves garlic, minced

1 tablespoon fresh
   sage, chopped

1 tablespoon fresh
   thyme, chopped

½ teaspoon salt

2 pounds ground turkey

1. Preheat the oven to 375°F. Line a baking sheet with parchment paper.

2. In a large skillet, heat the avocado oil over medium heat. Add the onion, celery, garlic, sage, thyme, and salt; sauté for 5 to 10 minutes until the veggies are soft, remove from heat, and let cool.

3. Place the ground turkey in a large bowl, and then add in the veggie mixture. Mix together until fully combined.

4. Form into 6 mini meatloaf shapes (about 4-by-2-by-2 inches) and place them on the baking sheet.

FOR THE CRANBERRY GLAZE

2 cups fresh cranberries

½ cup filtered water

1 tablespoon pure
   maple syrup

5. Bake for 30 minutes or until the internal temperature reaches 165°F. Meanwhile, make the cranberry glaze by combining the cranberries, water, and maple syrup in a small saucepan.

6. Bring the glaze to a slow boil over medium heat and then reduce the heat to low. Allow the sauce to simmer and thicken for 20 minutes, stirring often.

7. When fully cooked, remove the mini turkey loaves from the oven and top with the cranberry glaze.

Swaps: To lower the carb content, you can swap out the maple syrup for 1 tablespoon of erythritol if it has been successfully reintroduced.

Per Serving Calories: 297; Total Fat: 17g; Total Carbs: 8g; Fiber: 2g; Net Carbs: 6g; Protein: 27g MACROS · Fat: 52%; Protein: 38%; Carbs: 10%

LEMON AND HERB ROASTED CHICKEN

PREP TIME: 15 MINUTES | COOK TIME: 1 HOUR 30 MINUTES

AIP-Elimination Phase Compliant

SERVES 6

This classic roasted whole chicken comes out tender and flavorful every time. The key to getting a nice, crispy skin is to dry the outside of the chicken very well with paper towels. Once you have mastered roasting a whole chicken, you will want to make it again and again!

6 pound whole chicken, patted dry with innards removed

4 tablespoons coconut oil

1 tablespoon salt

1 lemon, cut in half

1 yellow onion, peeled and cut in half

1 head garlic, cut in half horizontally

20 fresh thyme sprigs

1. Preheat the oven to 425°F.

2. Place the chicken on a roasting pan or deep baking sheet.

3. Spread the coconut oil all over the inside and outside of the chicken, then season the same areas with salt.

4. Stuff the cavity of the chicken with the lemon, onion, garlic, and thyme.

5. Tie the drumsticks together with kitchen twine and tuck the wings under the body of the chicken.

6. Put the chicken in the oven and bake for about 90 minutes or until the internal temperature reaches 160°F.

7. Remove it from the oven and tent the chicken lightly with foil.

8. Allow the chicken to rest for 15 minutes. The internal temperature should reach 165°F.

9. Carve the chicken and serve.

Tips: Remove the packet of innards and drain the juice out from the inside of the chicken before patting the inside and outside dry. Use a meat thermometer to ensure the chicken has reached 165°F before serving.

Swaps: You can substitute the coconut oil for ghee or grass-fed butter if these have been successfully reintroduced. Before roasting the chicken, sprinkle it with ½ teaspoon of cracked black pepper if you have successfully reintroduced it.

Per Serving Calories: 559; Total Fat: 44g; Total Carbs: 0g; Fiber: 0g; Net Carbs: 0g; Protein: 38g MACROS · Fat: 71%; Protein: 29%; Carbs: 0%

GRILLED CHICKEN WITH DILL YOGURT SAUCE

PREP TIME: 5 MINUTES, PLUS 3 HOURS TO MARINATE |
COOK TIME: 40 MINUTES

AIP-Elimination Phase Compliant

SERVES 2

This grilled chicken dish is loaded with fresh lemon and herbs. We use coconut yogurt to make this marinade AIP-Elimination Phase Compliant, but it can also be made with plain Greek yogurt if you have successfully reintroduced dairy.

FOR THE MARINADE

4 skin-on chicken thighs

⅓ cup plain unsweetened
  Coconut Yogurt
  (page 178)

¼ red onion, thinly sliced

Juice and zest from
  ½ lemon

2 cloves garlic, minced

½ teaspoon salt

1 teaspoon dried oregano

1 tablespoon avocado oil

1½ tablespoons fresh
  parsley, chopped

1. Pat the chicken thighs dry and arrange them in a casserole dish.

2. In a medium bowl, combine the yogurt, red onion, lemon juice and zest, garlic, salt, oregano, avocado oil, and parsley. Pour it over the chicken thighs and coat fully.

3. Cover the casserole dish with plastic wrap and refrigerate for 3 to 5 hours.

4. When ready to cook, heat your grill or grill pan to medium heat.

5. Grill the chicken for 40 minutes (20 minutes on each side), or until the internal temperature reaches 165°F.

FOR THE SAUCE

⅓ cup plain unsweetened
   Coconut Yogurt
   (page 178)
1 clove garlic, minced
3 tablespoons fresh
   dill, chopped
1 teaspoon extra-virgin
   olive oil
1 teaspoon lemon juice
¼ teaspoon salt

6. Pour the coconut yogurt, garlic, dill, extra-virgin olive oil, lemon juice, and salt into a blender or food processor; process until smooth.

7. Serve in a small bowl for dipping or spoon it over the cooked chicken.

Tip: While grilling, check to make sure the chicken skin isn't turning black. If it is, turn the heat down slightly to ensure that the inside gets cooked and the skin is crispy and golden.

Per Serving Calories: 658; Total Fat: 54g; Total Carbs: 8g; Fiber: 2g; Net Carbs: 5g; Protein: 35g MACROS – Fat: 74%; Protein: 21%; Carbs: 5%

CRISPY OVEN-BAKED BUFFALO CHICKEN THIGHS

PREP TIME: 5 MINUTES | COOK TIME: 40 MINUTES

AIP-Reintroduction Phase: Dairy (blue cheese, ghee), Nightshades (cayenne pepper, hot pepper sauce, paprika), Non-AIP Spices (black pepper)

SERVES 4

Spicy and crisped to perfection, these buffalo chicken thighs make a delicious and satisfying dinner for any night of the week. We make our own buffalo sauce to avoid the soy and other additives that are found in most store-bought ones.

FOR THE CHICKEN

1 tablespoon aluminum-free
 baking powder

1 tablespoon salt

1 tablespoon paprika

¼ teaspoon black pepper

8 skin-on chicken thighs

¼ cup blue cheese
 crumbles (optional)

1. Preheat the oven to 375°F. Line a baking sheet with parchment paper.

2. In a small bowl, mix together the baking powder, salt, paprika, and pepper.

3. Pat the chicken thighs dry, place on the baking sheet and sprinkle the seasoning mixture over the chicken, coating all sides.

4. Bake for about 35 minutes or until the internal temperature reaches 165°F, then turn your oven to broil and broil for 3 to 5 minutes or until the skin is crisped.

FOR THE BUFFALO SAUCE

⅔ cup hot pepper sauce
  (like Frank's brand)

½ cup ghee

1½ teaspoons
  coconut aminos

¼ teaspoon cayenne pepper

¼ teaspoon garlic powder

¼ teaspoon paprika

5. In a small saucepan, prepare the buffalo sauce by heating all the ingredients over medium heat. Whisk until the ghee is melted and the sauce is fully combined.

6. Pour the sauce over the cooked chicken thighs, coating it on all sides.

7. Garnish with blue cheese crumbles (if using).

Tip: Putting salt and baking powder on the chicken dries the skin to help you achieve maximum crispness. We bake ours at 375°F and then broil them for the last 3 to 5 minutes, but you can also bake them at 400°F for about 35 minutes.

Per Serving Calories: 637; Total Fat: 56g; Total Carbs: 1g; Fiber: 0g; Net Carbs: 1g; Protein: 33g MACROS – Fat: 78%; Protein: 22%; Carbs: 0%

GRILLED CHICKEN SATAY

PREP TIME: 15 MINUTES, PLUS 3 HOURS TO MARINATE |
COOK TIME: 10 MINUTES

AIP-Reintroduction Phase: Nightshades (cayenne pepper, paprika),
Nuts (almond butter)

SERVES 6

Our Grilled Chicken Satay is perfect for cookouts or dinner parties, and can be served as a main dish or an appetizer. We marinate the chicken ahead of time, then grill it to perfection alongside a delicious dipping sauce!

FOR THE CHICKEN

2 pounds boneless, skinless
chicken thighs, cut into
1-inch pieces

2 tablespoons
coconut aminos

1 tablespoon fish sauce (like
Red Boat brand)

1 clove garlic, minced

1 teaspoon raw honey

1 tablespoon lime juice

1 teaspoon paprika

½ teaspoon turmeric

¼ cup fresh cilantro,
chopped, plus extra
for garnishing

2 scallions, chopped,
for garnish

TO MAKE THE CHICKEN

1. Pat the chicken thigh pieces dry and arrange them in a casserole dish.

2. In a medium bowl, combine the coconut aminos, fish sauce, garlic, honey, lime juice, paprika, turmeric, and cilantro. Pour the mixture over the chicken thighs and coat fully.

3. Cover the casserole dish with plastic wrap and refrigerate for 3 to 5 hours.

4. Heat your grill or grill pan to high.

5. Soak 12 wooden skewers in water for 15 minutes, then thread your chicken pieces evenly among each one.

6. Grill the chicken on all sides, turning it every few minutes, until the chicken reaches an internal temperature of 165°F, about 10 minutes. Remove it and cover it while you make your sauces.

7. Garnish with lime juice, chopped scallions, and chopped cilantro, and serve it with the dipping sauce.

FOR THE DIPPING SAUCE

1 teaspoon coconut oil

1 tablespoon grated
   ginger root

2 cloves garlic, minced

½ cup full-fat coconut milk

1 tablespoon
   coconut aminos

1 tablespoon lime juice

½ teaspoon cayenne pepper

3 tablespoons
   almond butter

TO MAKE THE DIPPING SAUCE

1. In a small saucepan, combine the coconut oil, ginger root, garlic, coconut milk, coconut aminos, lime juice, cayenne pepper, and almond butter over medium heat and stir until the almond butter is melted and all the ingredients are incorporated.

2. Pour the sauce into a small bowl.

Swap: Want to add some spicy kick? Add in 1 teaspoon of organic sriracha sauce to the dipping sauce, if it has been successfully reintroduced.

Per Serving: Calories: 309; Total Fat: 17g; Total Carbs: 4g; Fiber: 1g; Net Carbs: 3g; Protein: 35g MACROS - Fat: 50%; Protein: 45%; Carbs: 5%

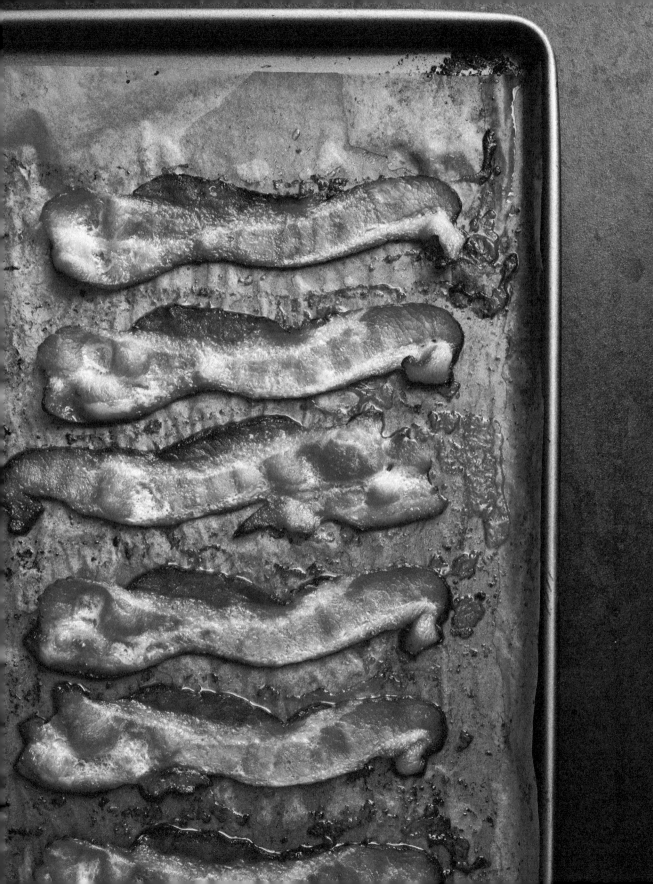

Chapter 8

BEEF AND PORK

SKIRT STEAK WITH CHIMICHURRI SAUCE

PREP TIME: 4 TO 8 HOURS | COOK TIME: 10 MINUTES

AIP-Elimination Phase Compliant

SERVES 2

This recipe results in perfectly tender beef every time. Marinate the steak and make the chimichurri ahead of time, then simply grill the meat up when you are ready to eat!

12-ounce skirt steak

2 tablespoons avocado oil

Juice from ½ lemon

1 clove garlic, minced

¼ teaspoon dried oregano

¼ teaspoon salt

½ cup Chimichurri Sauce
  (page 175)

1. Pat the steak dry and set in a casserole dish.

2. Combine the avocado oil, lemon juice, garlic, oregano, and salt in a bowl and pour over the steak to coat fully.

3. Cover the casserole dish with plastic wrap and refrigerate for 4 to 8 hours.

4. Heat your grill or grill pan to high.

5. Grill the steak for about 3 to 6 minutes on each side, or until the internal temperature reaches 125 to 130°F, then remove the steak from the grill to let rest for 5 minutes. The internal temperature should reach 130 to 135°F after resting.

6. Cut your steak against the grain. Drizzle with the Chimichurri Sauce.

Tip: Skirt steak is a thin cut of beef, so heat your grill to a very high temperature so that you develop a nice crust on the outside while keeping the inside medium rare.

Per Serving Calories: 746; Total Fat: 62g; Total Carbs: 3g; Fiber: 0g; Net Carbs: 3g; Protein: 44g MACROS - Fat: 75%; Protein: 24%; Carbs: 1%

GARLIC-STUDDED PRIME RIB
WITH THYME AU JUS

PREP TIME: 10 MINUTES | COOK TIME: 2 HOURS

AIP-Elimination Phase Compliant

SERVES 6 TO 8

Prime rib is one of our favorite cuts of beef to serve for a holiday dinner or special occasion. This recipe is AIP Elimination Phase Compliant and loaded with flavor.

6- to 7-pound bone-in
   prime rib

8 cloves garlic, thinly sliced

2 tablespoons salt

¼ cup red wine vinegar

4 cups Beef Bone Broth
   (store-bought or
   homemade, page 168)

1 tablespoon fresh
   thyme, chopped

1. Bring the prime rib to room temperature.

2. Preheat the oven to 350°F.

3. Make small slits in the prime rib and stuff each slit with a slice of garlic.

4. Season the prime rib liberally with salt and place it on a rack that is set inside a roasting pan.

5. Roast the prime rib for about 2 hours, or until the internal temperature reaches 130°F.

6. Remove the prime rib from the oven, transfer to a large platter, and tent it with foil to keep it warm while you make the au jus.

7. Place the roasting pan with the rack removed over two stove burners set to high heat.

8. Add the vinegar to the drippings in the pan and cook over high heat, scraping the bottom of the pan with a wooden spoon until the sauce is reduced.

CONTINUED

9. Add the beef bone broth and cook until it is reduced by half.

10. Whisk in the thyme and season the sauce with salt to taste.

11. Slice the meat to your desired thickness, plate, and pour the au jus over the beef.

Swaps: Prior to roasting the prime rib, sprinkle it with 2 teaspoons cracked black pepper if you have successfully reintroduced it. You can also substitute the red wine vinegar for ½ cup of dry red wine if you have successfully reintroduced alcohol.

Per Serving Calories: 897; Total Fat: 77g; Total Carbs: 0g; Fiber: 0g; Net Carbs: 0g; Protein: 51g MACROS - Fat: 77%; Protein: 23%; Carbs: 0%

GREEK MEATBALL LETTUCE WRAPS

PREP TIME: 10 MINUTES | COOK TIME: 20 MINUTES

AIP-Elimination Phase Compliant

SERVES 2

Full of fresh ingredients, these lettuce wraps are so flavorful and completely AIP-Elimination Phase Compliant. Feel free to serve over mixed greens as a salad rather than in a lettuce wrap.

½ pound ground lamb

2 tablespoons fresh parsley, finely chopped

½ teaspoon fresh mint, finely chopped

1 clove garlic, minced

1 teaspoon dried oregano

1 tablespoon avocado oil

2 Bibb lettuce leaves

1 avocado, sliced

2 tablespoons Cucumber Tzatziki (recipe on page 181)

1. Preheat the oven to 350°F. Line a baking sheet with parchment paper.

2. In a large bowl, mix the lamb, parsley, mint, garlic, and oregano until well combined.

3. Form the meat mixture into 1½-inch balls.

4. In medium-sized skillet, heat the avocado oil on high heat.

5. Place the meatballs in the skillet and sear on all sides for 5 to 10 minutes.

6. Transfer the seared meatballs to the baking sheet and bake for about 10 minutes or until the internal temperature reaches about 160°F.

7. Prepare the lettuce wraps by placing 2 to 3 meatballs inside each lettuce leaf and topping them with the avocado and Cucumber Tzatziki.

Tip: We love a good sear on these meatballs, but for easier cooking, you can skip the searing process and oven bake the meatballs at 425°F for about 20 minutes.

Per Serving Calories: 530; Total Fat: 48g; Total Carbs: 7g; Fiber: 5g; Net Carbs: 2g; Protein: 20g MACROS - Fat: 81%; Protein: 16%; Carbs: 5%

CILANTRO LIME TACO BOWLS

PREP TIME: 10 MINUTES | COOK TIME: 10 MINUTES

AIP-Elimination Phase Compliant

SERVES 2

These taco bowls are full of spiced ground beef, crisp romaine lettuce, sweet pickled onions, buttery avocados, and a tangy cilantro lime sauce! Best of all, this hearty meal comes together in just 20 minutes!

FOR THE TACO BOWL

2 tablespoons avocado oil

½ pound ground beef

½ teaspoon garlic powder

½ teaspoon onion powder

½ teaspoon dried oregano

6 cups romaine
  lettuce, chopped

¼ cup Grapefruit Red
  Onions (page 182)

2 avocados, diced

**FOR THE CILANTRO
LIME SAUCE**

¼ cup avocado oil

¼ cup lime juice

½ cup fresh cilantro

¼ teaspoon salt

1. In a large skillet, heat the avocado oil over medium heat.

2. Add the ground beef to the skillet and use a wooden spoon to break it into small crumbles.

3. Sprinkle the spices onto the meat and stir to combine.

4. Let the meat continue to cook for 10 minutes until no longer pink.

5. Make the Cilantro Lime Sauce by putting the avocado oil, lime juice, cilantro, and salt in a food processor or blender; process until smooth.

6. Divide the romaine lettuce among 4 bowls, top with the ground beef, red onions, avocado, and the Cilantro Lime Sauce.

Swaps: You can add 1 teaspoon of cumin and 1 teaspoon of cayenne pepper to the ground beef if they have been successfully reintroduced. You can also top the taco bowls with diced tomatoes, sour cream, or jalapenos if those foods have been successfully reintroduced.

Per Serving Calories: 840; Total Fat: 78g; Total Carbs: 18g; Fiber: 11g; Net Carbs: 7g; Protein: 27g MACROS - Fat: 81%; Protein: 12%; Carbs: 7%

FLANK STEAK WITH
SWEET HORSERADISH CREAM

PREP TIME: 10 MINUTES | COOK TIME: 10 MINUTES

AIP-Elimination Phase Compliant

SERVES 2

The star of this dish is our Sweet Horseradish Cream, which is fresh, spicy, and pairs wonderfully with tender flank steak. Flank steak is composed of long muscle fibers that create a natural grain in the meat. Be sure to slice it across the grain, otherwise the meat will be extremely chewy.

12-ounce flank steak

2 tablespoons avocado oil

¼ teaspoon salt

1 cup mixed greens

¼ red onion, thinly sliced

1 tablespoon capers

¼ cup Sweet Horseradish
    Cream (page 180)

1. Heat a grill or grill pan to high heat.

2. Pat the flank steak dry, then rub it with avocado oil and season with salt.

3. Grill the steak on both sides for a total of 6 to 8 minutes or until the internal temperature reaches 120 to 125°F.

4. Transfer the steak to a plate to let it rest for 5 to 10 minutes. The internal temperature should reach 130 to 135°F.

5. Slice the steak against the grain.

6. On a medium-size platter, assemble the dish by plating the mixed greens, then the red onion, sliced steak, capers, and Sweet Horseradish Cream.

Tip: To slice the steak against the grain, you first need to identify the direction that the muscle fibers are aligned. Once you identify this direction, slice your steak in the opposite direction, rather than parallel with it.

Swap: You can substitute skirt steak for the flank steak.

Per Serving Calories: 483; Total Fat: 31g; Total Carbs: 11g; Fiber: 3g; Net Carbs: 8g; Protein: 40g MACROS - Fat: 60%; Protein: 32%; Carbs: 8%

SLOW COOKER BARBACOA PULLED BEEF WITH CILANTRO CAULIFLOWER RICE

PREP TIME: 10 MINUTES | COOK TIME: 4 TO 8 HOURS

AIP-Elimination Phase Compliant

SERVES 6 TO 8

This barbacoa is extremely easy to make thanks to the slow cooker, and it pairs perfectly with cilantro cauliflower rice for a satisfying meal. If you have leftovers, store them in a sealed container in the refrigerator for up to 5 days.

FOR THE BARBACOA

5 pounds round roast

½ cup Beef Bone Broth (store-bought or homemade, page 168)

¼ cup lime juice, fresh squeezed

1 yellow onion, peeled and cut into 1-inch pieces

4 cloves garlic, minced

3 tablespoons apple cider vinegar

1 tablespoon salt

2 teaspoons dried oregano

TO MAKE THE BARBACOA

1. Put the round roast, beef broth, lime juice, onion, garlic, vinegar, salt, and oregano in 6-quart slow cooker.

2. Cook on low for 8 hours or high for 4 hours.

3. The beef is done when it easily falls apart with fork.

4. Shred the beef with two forks before serving.

FOR THE CILANTRO CAULIFLOWER RICE

2 heads cauliflower, chopped into florets

¼ cup avocado oil

4 cloves garlic, minced

2 teaspoons salt

Juice from 2 limes

½ cup fresh chopped cilantro, chopped

TO MAKE THE CAULIFLOWER RICE

1. Place the cauliflower florets in a food processor and pulse until the cauliflower resembles the size of rice. *(Depending on how big your food processor is, you may need to do this in batches.)*

2. In a large skillet, heat the avocado oil over medium heat.

3. Add the garlic and cook until soft, about 3 to 5 minutes.

4. Add the cauliflower "rice" and stir to combine.

5. Season with salt and cook for about 5 minutes, stirring frequently until the cauliflower softens.

6. Remove from heat and transfer to a serving bowl. Add in the lime juice and fresh cilantro and toss gently to combine.

Tips: Pair this dish with AIP toppings such as diced red onions, avocado, shredded purple cabbage, and our Cilantro Lime Sauce (page 134).

Swaps: Add 1 tablespoon cumin, 2 teaspoons cayenne pepper, and 2 teaspoons chili powder to the barbacoa if you have successfully reintroduced these spices.

Per Serving Calories: 562; Total Fat: 30g; Total Carbs: 8g; Fiber: 2g; Net Carbs: 6g; Protein: 65g MACROS - Fat: 48%; Protein: 46%; Carbs: 6%

GLAZED PORK TENDERLOIN

PREP TIME: 5 MINUTES | COOK TIME: 25 MINUTES

AIP-Elimination Phase Compliant

SERVES 6 TO 8

Pork tenderloins are a terrific option for when you want to cook up a hearty meal with little effort. The earthiness of the spice rub and the sweetness of the marinade come together to give you a dinner that is full of flavor.

2 pounds pork tenderloin

2 teaspoons salt

2 teaspoons fresh thyme

1½ teaspoons ground cinnamon

1½ teaspoons garlic powder

1 tablespoon fresh cilantro, chopped, for garnish (optional)

FOR THE GLAZE

2 tablespoons coconut aminos

1 tablespoon balsamic vinegar

1 teaspoon fish sauce (like Red Boat brand)

2 cloves garlic, minced

1. Preheat the oven to 375°F. Line a baking sheet with parchment paper.

2. Place the pork tenderloin on the baking sheet.

3. In a small bowl, mix together all the spices. Rub the spice mixture all over the pork.

4. Put the pork in the oven and bake for 15 minutes.

5. Meanwhile, prepare the glaze by mixing together the coconut aminos, vinegar, fish sauce, and garlic.

6. After 15 minutes, remove the pork from the oven and pour the glaze over it to fully coat.

7. Place the pork back in the oven to continue baking for another 10 minutes or until the internal temperature reaches 145°F.

8. Let the pork rest for 5 minutes, then slice and garnish with cilantro (if using).

Swap: Add 2 teaspoons cumin and 1 teaspoon cayenne pepper to the spice rub if you have successfully reintroduced these spices.

Per Serving Calories: 181; Total Fat: 5g; Total Carbs: 2g; Fiber: 0g; Net Carbs: 2g; Protein: 31g MACROS - Fat: 27%; Protein: 72%; Carbs: 1%

GRILLED BURGERS WITH BASIL AIOLI

PREP TIME: 10 MINUTES | COOK TIME: 10 MINUTES

AIP-Reintroduction Phase: Eggs & Egg-Based Sauces (mayo)

SERVES 4

Burgers can absolutely still be keto! All you need to do is get creative with substitutes for the standard bun. In this recipe, we use hearty portobello mushrooms, but you can also use lettuce leaves or even a collard green wrap.

FOR THE BURGERS

⅓ cup balsamic vinegar

½ cup avocado oil

2 cloves garlic, minced

4 Portobello mushroom caps, stems and gills removed, caps cleaned with damp paper towel

1 pound ground beef

1 avocado, sliced

FOR THE BASIL AIOLI

2 tablespoons avocado-oil mayonnaise (like Primal Kitchen brand)

2 tablespoons Basil Pesto (page 174)

1. In a small bowl, mix together the mayonnaise and Basil Pesto until well combined. Set aside.

2. In a large bowl, whisk together the balsamic vinegar, oil, and garlic.

3. Add the mushroom caps to the bowl and gently toss to coat fully in the marinade. Let sit for 10 minutes.

4. Meanwhile, form the ground beef into 4 patties.

5. Heat a grill or grill pan to medium heat.

6. Grill the burger patties and mushroom caps for 5 minutes on one side, then flip and grill for another 5 minutes.

7. Spread 1 tablespoon of Basil Aioli on each grilled mushroom cap, then place the burgers on top, followed by the sliced avocado.

Swap: Feel free to add your favorite burger toppings such as onions or even tomatoes and cheese if they have been successfully reintroduced.

Per Serving Calories: 613; Total Fat: 49g; Total Carbs: 10g; Fiber: 4g; Net Carbs: 6g; Protein: 33g MACROS - Fat: 72%; Protein: 22%; Carbs: 6%

CRACKED PEPPER FRIED PORK CHOPS

PREP TIME: 5 MINUTES | COOK TIME: 10 MINUTES

AIP-Reintroduction Phase: Eggs & Egg-Based Sauces (egg, mayo),
Nightshades (barbecue sauce, cayenne pepper, paprika),
Non-AIP Spices (black pepper)

SERVES 4

This recipe is perfect for those times you want something hearty and delicious, but don't have a lot of time to cook. Pork chops fry up quickly, which make them a go-to dinner option on a busy night.

FOR THE PORK CHOPS

1 cup coconut oil

2 (1.75-ounce) bags pork
    rinds (crushed)

2 tablespoons coconut flour

½ teaspoon cracked
    black pepper

½ teaspoon cayenne pepper

¼ teaspoon paprika

¼ teaspoon garlic powder

Pinch salt

1 egg

1 tablespoon full-fat
    coconut milk

4 pork chops, patted dry
    and seasoned with salt
    and cracked black pepper

1. In a large skillet, heat the coconut oil over medium heat.

2. In a shallow dish, combine the pork rinds, coconut flour, pepper, cayenne, paprika, garlic powder, and salt.

3. In another shallow dish, whisk together the egg and coconut milk.

4. Dip the pork into the egg mixture, then into the pork rind mixture, firmly pressing the crumbs into all sides.

5. Place the breaded pork chops in the skillet and fry for 3 to 4 minutes on each side or until they are golden brown and the internal temperature reaches 145°F.

6. Transfer the cooked pork chops to a wire rack to cool slightly.

FOR THE SAUCE

2 tablespoons Sweet
  Horseradish Cream
  (on page 180)
2 tablespoons sugar-free
  barbecue sauce (like
  Primal Kitchen brand)
2 tablespoons avocado-oil
  mayonnaise (like Primal
  Kitchen brand)
2 teaspoons fresh
  parsley, chopped, for
  garnish (optional)

7. In a small bowl, prepare the sauce by mixing together the Sweet Horseradish Cream, barbecue sauce, and mayonnaise.

8. Top the fried pork chops with the sauce and garnish with parsley (if using).

Tip: Crush your pork rinds by crunching them up with your hands in the bag or using a food processor.

Per Serving Calories: 469; Total Fat: 35g; Total Carbs: 6g; Fiber: 3g; Net Carbs: 3g; Protein: 33g MACROS - Fat: 68%; Protein: 27%; Carbs: 5%

GRILLED MOROCCAN SPICED LAMB

PREP TIME: 5 MINUTES | COOK TIME: 10 MINUTES

AIP-Reintroduction Phase: Nightshades (cayenne pepper),
Non-AIP Spices (cumin, cardamom, black pepper)

SERVES 4

Lamb is an excellent source of protein and also full of nutrients like iron, zinc, selenium, and vitamin B12. In this recipe, we pair lamb chops with mint to create a delicious and cohesive dish. You'll be amazed at how quickly it comes together with very little effort!

½ teaspoon cumin

¼ teaspoon cardamom

¼ teaspoon ground ginger

¼ teaspoon cayenne pepper

¼ teaspoon
  ground cinnamon

¼ teaspoon salt

¼ teaspoon garlic powder

⅛ teaspoon black pepper

8 lamb chops (about
  2 pounds)

1 tablespoon fresh
  cilantro, chopped, for
  garnish (optional)

1. In a small bowl, mix together the cumin, cardamom, ginger, cayenne, cinnamon, salt, garlic powder, and pepper.

2. Sprinkle both sides of the lamb chops with the spice mixture.

3. Heat your grill or grill pan to high heat and grill the lamb for 2 to 3 minutes on each side or until the internal temperature reaches 130 to 135°F.

4. Garnish with fresh cilantro (if using) and serve.

Tips: Make extra Moroccan spice blend and store in a sealed container at room temperature for up to 6 months.

Per Serving Calories: 354; Total Fat: 24g; Total Carbs: 1g; Fiber: 0g; Net Carbs: 1g; Protein: 31g MACROS - Fat: 62%; Protein: 37%; Carbs: 1%

SESAME SLAW WITH GROUND PORK

PREP TIME: 5 MINUTES | COOK TIME: 15 MINUTES

AIP-Reintroduction Phase: Nightshades (sriracha), Non-AIP Spices
(black pepper), Seeds (sesame oil)

SERVES 4

This Asian-inspired dish is our version of an "egg roll in a bowl." We have taken all the flavors of your favorite egg roll and turned them into a quick and easy low-carb dish, without the added sugars and grain-filled wrapper.

2 tablespoons sesame oil

½ cup yellow onion, diced

2 cloves garlic, minced

2 teaspoons grated
  ginger root

1½ pounds ground pork

1 teaspoon salt

¼ teaspoon black pepper

1 (12 ounce) bag of
  coleslaw mix

1 tablespoon sriracha sauce

3 tablespoons
  coconut aminos

1 tablespoon white
  wine vinegar

1. In large skillet, heat the sesame oil over medium heat.

2. Add in the onion, garlic, and ginger and sauté for 2 to 3 minutes. Then add in the pork, salt, and pepper.

3. Continue cooking for 10 minutes. Once the pork is just about done cooking, stir in the slaw, sriracha, coconut aminos, and vinegar.

4. Cook for an additional 3 to 5 minutes until the slaw has softened slightly but is still crisp.

Tip: Opt for an organic sriracha sauce that doesn't include any additives.

Per Serving Calories: 539; Total Fat: 43g; Total Carbs: 8g; Fiber: 3g; Net Carbs: 5g; Protein: 30g MACROS - Fat: 72%; Protein: 22%; Carbs: 6%

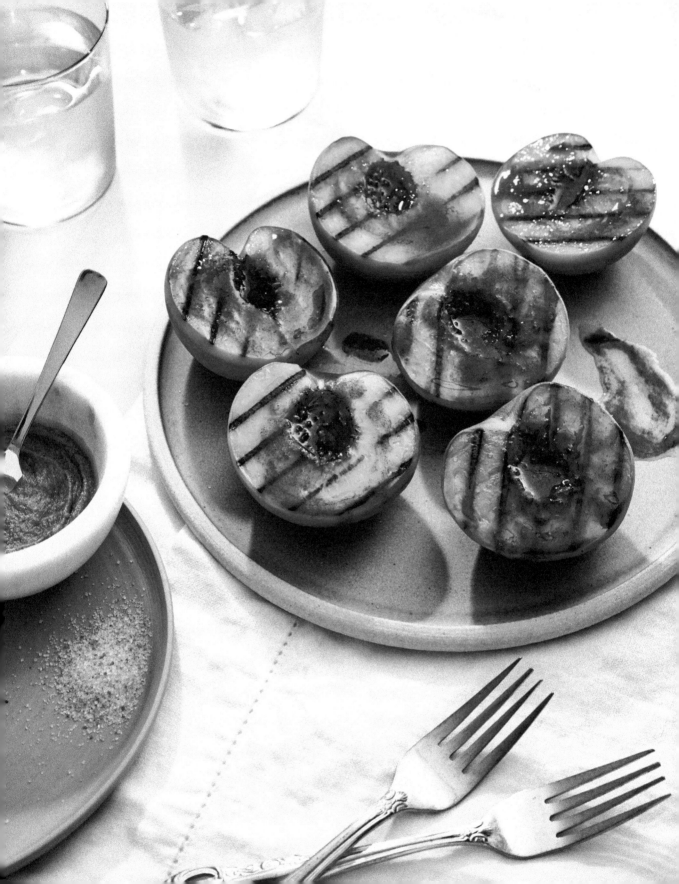

Chapter 9

DESSERTS

VANILLA PANNA COTTA

PREP TIME: 5 MINUTES, PLUS 4 HOURS TO CHILL | COOK TIME: 10 MINUTES

AIP-Elimination Phase Compliant

SERVES 4

This crave-worthy dessert is a delicious way to sneak beef gelatin into your diet. Gelatin can help ease joint pain, aid in digestive function, and improve skin health.

1 (14 ounce) can full-fat coconut milk

Pinch salt

4 teaspoons raw honey, divided

½ teaspoon gluten-free vanilla extract

1 tablespoon beef gelatin powder (like Great Lakes or Vital Proteins brand)

1. In a medium saucepan, heat the coconut milk, salt, and 3 teaspoons of honey over medium heat for 5 minutes, or until the honey is dissolved.

2. Stir in the vanilla and then turn off the heat.

3. Slowly whisk in the gelatin powder, making sure to break apart any clumps.

4. Grease three ramekins with coconut oil.

5. Pour the mixture evenly into the ramekins.

6. Refrigerate for 4 hours or until mixture has set firmly.

7. Before serving, dip the ramekins in warm water for 10 seconds to loosen the panna cotta from the dish.

8. Place a plate upside down on top of the ramekin, then flip it over. The panna cotta should come out onto the plate.

9. Drizzle the remaining 1 teaspoon of honey over the 4 panna cottas before serving.

Tip: Make sure to use gluten-free vanilla extract, as grain alcohol is often used in vanilla extract.

Swap: To lower the carb content, you can swap out the 3 teaspoons of honey for 3 teaspoons of erythritol if it has been successfully reintroduced. We recommend still drizzling 1 teaspoon of honey over the panna cottas before serving.

Per Serving Calories: 237; Total Fat: 21g; Total Carbs: 8g; Fiber: 0g; Net Carbs: 8g; Protein: 4g MACROS · Fat: 79%; Protein: 8%; Carbs: 13%

ROASTED STRAWBERRIES WITH WHIPPED CREAM

PREP TIME: 10 MINUTES, PLUS 30 MINUTES TO CHILL | COOK TIME: 10 MINUTES

AIP-Elimination Phase Compliant

SERVES 6

Strawberries are the perfect keto-friendly way to satisfy your sweet tooth. By roasting them in the oven, the strawberries caramelize and develop a concentrated sweetness as they break down and release their juices. Top these warm strawberries with coconut whipped cream for the perfect dessert. For best results, chill the bowl and electric mixer beaters in the freezer for at least an hour before making the coconut whipped cream.

1 cup coconut cream, refrigerated overnight

2 teaspoons raw honey

3 cups strawberries, stems removed and halved

2 teaspoons gluten-free vanilla extract

1. In a medium bowl, use an electric mixer to beat together the coconut cream and honey for 5 to 10 minutes or until fluffy.

2. Refrigerate the whipped cream for 30 minutes to allow it to firm up more.

3. Preheat the oven to 375°F. Line a baking sheet with parchment paper.

4. In another medium bowl, toss the strawberries and vanilla together.

5. Spread the strawberries in a single layer on the baking sheet and bake for 10 minutes.

6. Top the roasted strawberries with the chilled whipped cream.

Swap: To lower the carb content, you can swap out the honey for 2 teaspoons of confectioner erythritol if it has been successfully reintroduced.

Per Serving Calories: 166; Total Fat: 12g; Total Carbs: 11g; Fiber: 3g; Net Carbs: 8g; Protein: 2g MACROS · Fat: 71%; Protein: 4%; Carbs: 25%

GRILLED SWEET PEACHES

PREP TIME: 5 MINUTES | COOK TIME: 15 MINUTES

AIP-Elimination Phase Compliant

SERVES 6

Nothing is better than enjoying a perfectly ripe peach fresh from your local farmers' market. Except one thing—grilling that peach in order to bring out its natural juices and intensify its sweetness!

2 tablespoons coconut oil

2 teaspoons honey

½ teaspoon ground cinnamon

3 peaches, cut in half and pits removed

½ teaspoon salt

1. Combine the coconut oil, honey, and cinnamon in a small bowl.
2. Heat your grill or grill pan to medium-high heat.
3. Grill your peaches for 7 to 8 minutes on each side.
4. Top each grilled peach half with an even amount of the coconut mixture and sprinkle with a pinch of salt.

Tip: A whole peach has around 12 net carbs, so stick with half a peach as a serving size.

Swaps: To lower the carb content, you can swap out the honey for 2 teaspoons of confectioner erythritol if it has been successfully reintroduced.

Per Serving Calories: 75; Total Fat: 5g; Total Carbs: 9g; Fiber: 1g; Net Carbs: 8g; Protein: 1g MACROS - Fat: 54%; Protein: 3%; Carbs: 43%

COCONUT LIME MACAROONS

PREP TIME: 5 MINUTES | COOK TIME: 10 TO 12 MINUTES

AIP-Elimination Phase Compliant

MAKES 10 TO 12 MACAROONS

Coconut and lime are a classic pairing. These macaroons take those flavors and combine them into an indulgent AIP-Elimination Phase Compliant cookie that has amazing flavor and texture. No one will know that they are low-carb and anti-inflammatory!

1½ cups unsweetened shredded coconut

½ cup coconut butter (also called manna)

2 tablespoons collagen peptides powder

2 tablespoons coconut flour

1 tablespoon raw honey

1 tablespoon lime juice

1½ teaspoons lime zest, plus extra for garnish

1. Preheat the oven to 350°F. Line a baking sheet with parchment paper.

2. Mix all the ingredients in a medium bowl, using your hands to break apart any coconut butter clumps.

3. Roll the mixture into 1½-inch balls and place them on the baking sheet.

4. Bake the cookies for 10 to 12 minutes or until the outsides start to brown.

5. Remove them from the oven and garnish each macaroon with extra lime zest.

Tip: If your dough is crumbly, add in more coconut butter 1 teaspoon at a time until the dough stays compact.

Swaps: To lower the carb content, you can swap out the honey for 2 teaspoons of erythritol if it has been successfully reintroduced.

Per Serving Calories: 164; Total Fat: 15g; Total Carbs: 9g; Fiber: 5g; Net Carbs: 4g; Protein: 3g MACROS - Fat: 75%; Protein: 5%; Carbs: 20%

RASPBERRY MAPLE SOFT SERVE

PREP TIME: 5 MINUTES, PLUS OPTIONAL CHILLING

AIP-Elimination Phase Compliant

SERVES 4

Whip up this luscious soft-serve treat whenever you want something cold and sweet. It comes together quickly with only 3 ingredients! Simply adjust the recipe if you are serving more people.

1 cup coconut cream, refrigerated overnight

1 cup frozen raspberries

1 teaspoon pure maple syrup

1. Put the coconut cream, raspberries, and maple syrup in a blender. Process until smooth and creamy.

2. Scoop into a bowl and serve immediately if you like a soft-serve texture.

3. If you prefer a harder ice cream texture, you can place the blended mixture into a sealed container and freeze for an hour. Stir the mixture halfway to remove any hard or frozen sections.

Tips: If you don't have coconut cream available, place a can of full-fat coconut milk in the refrigerator overnight and simply skim the solid white cream that rises to the top of a can.

Swaps: To lower the carb content, you can swap out the maple syrup for 1 teaspoon of erythritol or 4 drops liquid stevia extract if these have been successfully reintroduced.

Per Serving Calories: 241; Total Fat: 21g; Total Carbs: 10g; Fiber: 4g; Net Carbs: 6g; Protein: 3g MACROS · Fat: 78%; Protein: 5%; Carbs: 17%

ULTRA-SOFT PUMPKIN CHOCOLATE CHIP BARS

PREP TIME: 5 MINUTES | COOK TIME: 30 MINUTES

AIP-Reintroduction Phase: Dairy (ghee), Eggs & Egg-Based Sauces, Keto Sweeteners (erythritol), Non-AIP spices (pumpkin pie spice), Seeds (chocolate)

MAKES 15 BARS

Although these indulgent bars feature pumpkin, you will want to make them any time of the year! They are super moist and have an almost fudgy consistency, which makes them irresistible.

½ cup ghee, melted

1 egg

¾ cup pumpkin purée

½ cup packed granular erythritol (like Swerve brand)

1 tablespoon gluten-free vanilla extract

2 teaspoons ground cinnamon

1 teaspoon pumpkin pie spice

1¼ cups almond flour

1 cup 85-percent dark chocolate chips or sugar-free chocolate chips (like Lily's brand)

1. Preheat the oven to 350°F. Line an 8-by-11-inch baking dish with parchment paper.

2. In a large bowl, mix together the ghee and egg, followed by the pumpkin purée and erythritol.

3. Add the vanilla extract, cinnamon, pumpkin pie spice, and the almond flour. Mix well until the flour is fully incorporated.

4. Fold in the chocolate chips.

5. Pour the batter into the baking dish and bake for 30 to 35 minutes or until a wooden toothpick inserted in the middle comes out clean.

6. Allow it to cool before slicing it into bars.

Tip: Make sure to use gluten-free vanilla extract, as grain alcohol is often used in vanilla extract.

Swaps: If you can find the golden granular erythritol, use it instead as it provides a deeper flavor. Also, feel free to swap out the ghee for 1 stick of grass-fed butter.

Per Serving Calories: 150; Total Fat: 12g; Total Carbs: 9g; Fiber: 2g; Net Carbs: 7g; Protein: 2g MACROS · Fat: 71%; Protein: 6%; Carbs: 23%

LEMON SNOWBALL COOKIES

PREP TIME: 5 MINUTES | COOK TIME: 20 MINUTES

AIP-Reintroduction Phase: Keto Sweeteners (erythritol)

MAKES 12 COOKIES

With a vibrant flavor and soft texture, these bite-sized lemon cookies are delicate and delicious. They are called Snowball Cookies because they are rolled in confectioner erythritol. Look for non-GMO versions of the keto-friendly sweetener in your grocery store or online. If you can't find confectioner erythritol, make your own by pulsing the granular erythritol in your food processor for 5 to 10 minutes until powdery.

½ cup coconut flour

2 tablespoons collagen peptides powder

¼ teaspoon baking soda

¼ cup coconut oil, melted

¼ cup granular erythritol (like Swerve brand)

Dash salt

½ tablespoon beef gelatin powder (like Great Lakes or Vital Proteins brand)

3 tablespoons filtered water, divided

2 tablespoons lemon juice

2 teaspoons lemon zest

½ teaspoon gluten-free vanilla extract

6 tablespoons confectioner erythritol (like Swerve brand), divided

1. Preheat the oven to 325°F. Line a baking sheet with parchment paper.

2. In a medium bowl, mix together the coconut flour, collagen, baking soda, coconut oil, erythritol, and salt.

3. Add the gelatin to a small bowl and bloom it by adding 1 tablespoon of lukewarm water to the gelatin, whisking vigorously, followed by 2 tablespoons of hot water, whisking vigorously again.

4. Immediately pour the gelatin mixture into the dough mixture, followed by the lemon juice, zest, and vanilla extract. Stir to incorporate well.

5. Roll the dough into 1½-inch balls, then gently roll them in 3 tablespoons of confectioner erythritol.

6. Place the balls on the baking sheet.

7. Bake the cookies for about 18 minutes or until they start to turn golden.

8. Let the cookies cool slightly, then roll them again in the remaining 3 tablespoons of confectioner erythritol.

Tips: Double the recipe if you are serving a larger crowd. Add ½ teaspoon of lemon extract for a more intense lemon flavor. Make sure to use gluten-free vanilla extract, as grain alcohol is often used in vanilla extract.

Swaps: You can substitute the coconut oil for ghee or grass-fed butter if these have been successfully reintroduced.

Per Serving Calories: 83; Total Fat: 6g; Total Carbs: 6g; Fiber: 4g; Net Carbs: 2g; Protein: 2g MACROS - Fat: 62%; Protein: 10%; Carbs: 28%

CRÈME BRÛLÉE

AIP-Reintroduction Phase: Eggs & Egg-Based Sauces,
Keto Sweeteners (erythritol)

SERVES 6 TO 8

It's completely possible to make a tasty low-carb Crème Brûlée. This dish is smooth and custardy and has a perfectly crisped top layer. With only 4 ingredients, this fancy dessert is surprisingly easy to make!

4 cups coconut cream

¾ cup granular erythritol (like Swerve brand), divided

6 large egg yolks

2 teaspoons gluten-free vanilla extract

1. Preheat the oven to 325°F.

2. In a medium saucepan, bring the coconut cream to a boil, remove it from the heat, and stir in the vanilla extract. Cover the pan and let it sit for 15 minutes.

3. In a medium bowl, whisk together 6 tablespoons erythritol and the egg yolks.

4. Slowly add the cream mixture to the yolk mixture, stirring continually.

5. Pour the custard mixture into 6 to 8 ramekins.

6. Place the ramekins in a large roasting pan. Pour hot water into the side of the pan so that the water comes halfway up the sides of the ramekins.

7. Bake for 40 to 45 minutes or until the custard is set but still jiggly.

8. Transfer the ramekins to the refrigerator for 2 hours.

9. Remove the ramekins from the refrigerator and allow them to rest and come to room temperature, about 30 minutes.

10. Sprinkle the remaining erythritol evenly over the tops of each custard.

11. Use a torch to melt the erythritol on top. Wait until the top shell hardens, then serve. If you don't have a kitchen torch, you can also broil the custards in the oven for 3 to 5 minutes or until the tops start to brown.

Tip: Make sure to use gluten-free vanilla extract, as grain alcohol is often used in vanilla extract.

Swap: You can substitute the coconut cream for an equal amount of heavy cream if you have successfully reintroduced dairy.

Per Serving Calories: 436; Total Fat: 45g; Total Carbs: 8g; Fiber: 3g; Net Carbs: 5g; Protein: 6g MACROS – Fat: 87%; Protein: 5%; Carbs: 8%

COCONUT CINNAMON BARS

PREP TIME: 5 MINUTES | COOK TIME: 5 MINUTES, PLUS 2 HOURS SET TIME

AIP-Reintroduction Phase: Eggs & Egg-Based Sauces,
Keto Sweeteners (erythritol)

SERVES 8

Make these delicious coconut cinnamon bars on the weekend, and you will have the perfect on-the-go treat ready for you all week!

1 (7 ounce) bag unsweetened shredded coconut

6 tablespoons granular erythritol (like Swerve brand)

½ cup filtered water

1 teaspoon gluten-free vanilla extract

2 teaspoons ground cinnamon

¼ cup collagen peptides powder

½ cup confectioner erythritol (like Swerve brand)

2⅓ tablespoons full-fat coconut milk

1. Preheat the oven to 350°F.

2. On a baking sheet, spread out the shredded coconut in an even layer, and bake for 3 to 5 minutes or until the coconut just starts to turn golden.

3. In a medium saucepan, mix the erythritol and water over medium heat and let it thicken and bubble for 5 minutes.

4. Add the vanilla extract and cinnamon, and stir. Turn off the heat.

5. Slowly whisk in the collagen peptides, making sure to break apart any clumps.

6. Stir in the toasted coconut.

7. Line a 9-by-13-inch casserole dish with parchment paper.

8. Press the coconut mixture into the dish firmly and allow to cool. Set for 2 hours.

9. Once cooled and firmed, cut the coconut mixture into 8 evenly sized bars.

10. In a small bowl, stir together the confectioner erythritol and coconut milk; if needed, add a bit more coconut milk until you reach your desired icing consistency.

11. Drizzle or pipe your icing onto each bar in diagonal stripes. Allow the icing to set before serving.

Tips: Make sure to use gluten-free vanilla extract, as grain alcohol is often used in vanilla extract. Store the bars in a sealed container at room temperature for up to 7 days.

Swap: If you cannot find confectioner erythritol, you can make your own by pulsing the granular erythritol in your food processor for 5 to 10 minutes or until powdery.

Per Serving: Calories: 293; Total Fat: 30g; Total Carbs: 8g; Fiber: 4g; Net Carbs: 4g; Protein: 6g MACROS - Fat: 84%; Protein: 7%; Carbs: 9%

CINNAMON POPOVERS WITH COCONUT STREUSEL

PREP TIME: 5 MINUTES | COOK TIME: 20 MINUTES

AIP-Reintroduction Phase: Eggs & Egg-Based Sauces,
Keto Sweeteners (erythritol)

SERVES 12

These popovers are full of warm cinnamon flavors and have an incredibly fluffy texture, making them the perfect breakfast or brunch option to serve for a crowd. Bonus: They take only 20 minutes to make and taste incredible straight out of the oven.

FOR THE POPOVERS

¼ cup coconut oil

3 teaspoons ground
   cinnamon, divided

6 eggs

½ cup full-fat coconut milk

¼ cup almond flour

3 tablespoons granular
   erythritol (like
   Swerve brand)

1. Preheat the oven to 400°F.

2. In a saucepan, melt the coconut oil and 1 teaspoon of ground cinnamon over medium heat.

3. In a 12-well muffin tin, evenly pour the melted coconut oil mixture into each well.

4. Place the muffin tin in the oven and heat for 3 minutes, or until the oil sizzles.

5. Mix the eggs, coconut milk, almond flour, the remaining 2 teaspoons of ground cinnamon, and the erythritol together in a medium bowl.

6. Evenly pour the egg mixture into each well.

7. Immediately place the muffin tin back in the oven, and bake for 10 minutes or until the popovers have significantly risen and are golden brown.

FOR THE TOPPING

3 tablespoons coconut oil

3 tablespoons granular erythritol (like Swerve brand)

3 tablespoons almond flour

2 teaspoons ground cinnamon

¼ cup unsweetened shredded coconut

8. While the popovers are baking, make the topping by mixing the coconut oil, erythritol, almond flour, cinnamon, and shredded coconut in a small bowl.

9. Remove the muffin tin from the oven and top each popover evenly with the crumb mixture.

10. Place the popovers back in the oven for an additional 3 to 5 minutes until the shredded coconut is golden brown.

Tip: Resist the urge to open your oven during baking! Doing so will reduce the amount your popovers rise. Instead, turn on your oven light and look through the oven door. The popovers will deflate once out of the oven. This is to be expected.

Per Serving Calories: 143; Total Fat: 14g; Total Carbs: 1g; Fiber: 0g; Net Carbs: 1g; Protein: 4g MACROS - Fat: 86%; Protein: 10%; Carbs: 4%

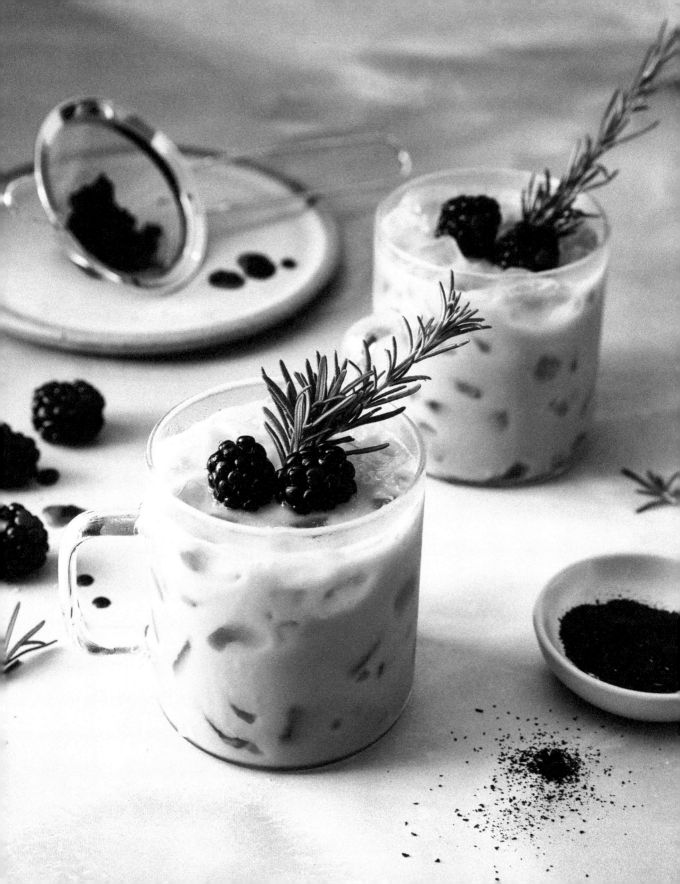

Chapter 10

BEVERAGES AND BROTHS

HEALING GOLDEN MILK

PREP TIME: 5 MINUTES | COOK TIME: 5 MINUTES

AIP-Elimination Phase Compliant

SERVES 1

Turmeric and its main active ingredient, curcumin, have powerful anti-inflammatory effects on the body. This Healing Golden Milk is especially comforting on a cold winter's day. The turmeric, ginger, and cinnamon are a classic combination and provide a warming flavor.

1½ cups full-fat
   coconut milk
1 teaspoon ground turmeric
⅛ teaspoon ground ginger
⅛ teaspoon ground
   cinnamon
2 teaspoons coconut oil
1 teaspoon raw
   honey (optional)

1. In a saucepan, combine the coconut milk, turmeric, ginger, cinnamon, coconut oil, and honey (if using) over medium heat and whisk to combine.

2. Remove from the heat when the liquid is hot, but not boiling.

3. Pour into a large mug and serve.

Swaps: Add a pinch of black pepper for extra anti-inflammatory benefits if you have successfully reintroduced it. To lower the carb content, you can swap out the honey for 1 teaspoon of erythritol or 4 drops liquid stevia extract if these have been successfully reintroduced.

Per Serving Calories: 744; Total Fat: 76g; Total Carbs: 9g; Fiber: 0g; Net Carbs: 9g; Protein: 7g MACROS – Fat: 92%; Protein: 3%; Carbs: 5%

ANTI-INFLAMMATORY
APPLE CIDER VINEGAR TONIC

PREP TIME: 5 MINUTES

AIP-Elimination Phase Compliant

SERVES 1

Apple cider vinegar has many detoxifying and beneficial properties, including improving digestion, fighting kidney and bladder problems, and aiding in weight loss. Make sure you get the apple cider vinegar with "the mother," which are naturally occurring enzymes within the vinegar that contain most of the healing properties.

2 cups filtered water

1 tablespoon apple
cider vinegar

1 teaspoon grated
ginger root

1 teaspoon raw
honey (optional)

1. Pour the water, apple cider vinegar, ginger root, and honey (if using) into a large glass. Stir together until combined.

2. Fill the glass with ice and serve immediately.

Tips: Using slightly warmed water will help to dissolve the honey. Add some additional flavors to your drink by stirring in lemon juice or muddling in fresh berries or herbs.

Swaps: To lower the carb content, you can swap out the honey for 1 teaspoon of erythritol or 4 drops liquid stevia extract if these have been successfully reintroduced.

Per Serving Calories: 12; Total Fat: 0g; Total Carbs: 3g; Fiber: 0g; Net Carbs: 3g; Protein: 0g MACROS - Fat: 0%; Protein: 0%; Carbs: 100%

THYME-INFUSED LEMONADE

PREP TIME: 5 MINUTES | COOK TIME: 15 MINUTES

AIP-Elimination Phase Compliant

SERVES 1

Lemons are high in vitamin C, which has been shown to boost immunity, prevent aging, and aid in repairing cells and tissues. This drink is a twist on the classic version of lemonade and is perfect for serving at brunches, showers, and cookouts.

1½ cups filtered
   water, divided
1 teaspoon coconut sugar
2 sprigs thyme
¼ cup lemon juice

1. In a small saucepan, combine ½ cup water and the coconut sugar over medium heat.

2. Bring the mixture to a simmer and stir until the coconut sugar is dissolved.

3. Add the thyme and lemon juice and continue to gently simmer for 1 minute.

4. Remove the pan from the heat and let it sit for 10 minutes.

5. Remove the thyme sprigs.

6. In a large glass filled with ice, stir in the remaining 1 cup water and the lemon thyme mixture.

Tip: This recipe can easily be modified to serve a large crowd. Simply put all the ingredients into a large pitcher before serving. For a beautiful presentation, garnish each glass with a lemon slice and a sprig of thyme.

Swap: To lower the carb content, you can swap out the coconut sugar for 1 teaspoon of erythritol if it has been successfully reintroduced.

Per Serving Calories: 28; Total Fat: 0g; Total Carbs: 7g; Fiber: 0g; Net Carbs: 7g; Protein: 0g MACROS – Fat: 0%; Protein: 6%; Carbs: 94%

CUCUMBER MINT SPRITZER

PREP TIME: 5 MINUTES

AIP-Elimination Phase Compliant

SERVES 1

This spritzer contains two incredible flavors—cucumber and mint. Cucumber is high in fiber, potassium, and vitamin C. Mint contains rosmarinic, an antioxidant found to relieve allergy symptoms. Together these flavors make a light and refreshing drink that will soon be your go-to beverage of choice. Use a spiralizer to create thin cucumber ribbons, or use a vegetable peeler to make long strands.

2 cucumber ribbons or
   long strands

2 tablespoons mint leaves

1½ cups sparkling water

1. In a large glass, muddle the cucumber ribbons and the mint leaves.

2. Add in your desired amount of ice, then pour in the sparkling water.

Swaps: To make this a refreshing cocktail, add in ½ cup dry white wine or 2 ounces vodka if you have successfully reintroduced alcohol.

Per Serving Calories: 0; Total Fat: 0g; Total Carbs: 0g; Fiber: 0g; Net Carbs: 0g; Protein: 0g MACROS – Fat: 0%; Protein: 0%; Carbs: 0%

CHICKEN BONE BROTH

PREP TIME: 5 MINUTES | COOK TIME: 11 TO 27 HOURS

AIP-Elimination Phase Compliant

SERVES 12

The healing benefits of drinking bone broth are numerous and include improved digestion and immune health. The long cooking time ensures the highest level of nutrient extraction from the bones as possible. We recommend drinking a cup a day as part of your healing journey.

2 to 3 pounds raw
chicken bones

4 cups roughly chopped
onion, celery, and carrots
(1⅓ cups each veggie)

1 tablespoon apple
cider vinegar

2 bay leaves

1 teaspoon salt

1. Preheat the oven to 350°F.

2. Roast the chicken bones for 30 minutes in a large roasting pan.

3. Transfer the bones to a large pot. Add the vegetables, vinegar, bay leaves, and salt.

4. Fill the pot with enough filtered water so that the bones are covered by about 1 inch. Bring the broth to a boil, then reduce the heat to a simmer and cover.

5. After 2 hours, use a slotted spoon to skim off any impurities that floated to the surface and discard.

6. Continue to cook the broth on the lowest heat for 8 to 24 hours.

7. Remove the broth from the heat and let it cool slightly for 20 minutes or so.

8. Carefully use a strainer to remove the bones and vegetables. Store your broth in sealed containers in the refrigerator for up to 5 days or freeze it for future use.

Tips: Try to use chicken feet, necks, and backs, as these have more gelatin. Make sure your broth isn't cooking at too high of a temperature or your broth may take on a cloudy appearance.

Per Serving Calories: 40; Total Fat: 0g; Total Carbs: 0g; Fiber: 0g; Net Carbs: 0g; Protein: 10g MACROS – Fat: 0%; Protein: 100%; Carbs: 0%

BEEF BONE BROTH

PREP TIME: 5 MINUTES | COOK TIME: 11 TO 27 HOURS

AIP-Elimination Phase Compliant

SERVES 12

Beef Bone Broth is a staple in our kitchens and is used for the base of many of our soups. It is gut-healing, nourishing, and has a rich, incredible depth of flavor.

2 to 3 pounds raw
   beef bones

4 cups roughly chopped
   onion, celery, and carrots
   (1⅓ cups each veggie)

1 tablespoon apple
   cider vinegar

2 bay leaves

1 teaspoon salt

1. Preheat the oven to 350°F.

2. Roast the beef bones for 30 minutes in a large roasting pan.

3. Transfer the bones to a large pot. Add the vegetables, vinegar, bay leaves, and salt.

4. Fill the pot with enough filtered water so that the bones are covered by about 1 inch. Bring the broth to a boil, then reduce the heat to a simmer and cover.

5. After 2 hours, use a slotted spoon to skim off any impurities that floated to the surface and discard.

6. Cook the broth on the lowest heat for 8 to 24 hours.

7. Remove the broth from the heat and let it cool slightly for 20 minutes or so.

8. Carefully use a strainer to remove the bones and vegetables. Store your broth in sealed containers in the refrigerator for up to 5 days or freeze it for future use.

Tips: Look for high-quality bones from grass-fed cattle. You can buy beef bones from your local butcher and/or ask them to order some for you. To make a broth with the most collagen, try to use feet, knuckles, necks, and backs.

Per Serving Calories: 40; Total Fat: 0g; Total Carbs: 0g; Fiber: 0g; Net Carbs: 0g; Protein: 10g MACROS – Fat: 0%; Protein: 100%; Carbs: 0%

DAIRY-FREE HOT CHOCOLATE

PREP TIME: 5 MINUTES | COOK TIME: 5 MINUTES

AIP-Reintroduction Phase: Nightshades (cayenne),
Nuts (almond milk), Seeds (cacao/cocoa)

SERVES 1

This dairy-free hot chocolate is rich, creamy, and oh-so-good for those cold nights when you are craving something comforting. We also provided optional add-ins that will upgrade the flavor profile even more!

1 cup unsweetened
  almond milk

2 tablespoons cacao or
  cocoa powder

1 tablespoon
  granular erythritol

⅛ teaspoon gluten-free
  vanilla extract

Pinch salt

OPTIONAL ADD-INS:

*For Peppermint Hot
  Chocolate:* 1 to 2 drops of
  peppermint extract

For Mexican Hot Chocolate:
  ⅛ teaspoon ground
  cinnamon and a small
  pinch of cayenne pepper

1. In a small saucepan, heat the almond milk, cacao/cocoa powder, erythritol, vanilla, and salt and add-in of choice (if using) on medium heat, whisking along the way until all the ingredients are combined.

2. Remove from the heat when the liquid is hot, but not boiling.

3. Pour into a large mug and serve.

Tips: Look for almond milk brands with no additives. The only ingredients on the food label should be almonds and water. Make sure to use gluten-free vanilla extract, as grain alcohol is often used in vanilla extract.

Swaps: Substitute the almond milk with an equal amount of coconut milk if you prefer the taste.

Per Serving Calories: 72; Total Fat: 4g; Total Carbs: 6g; Fiber: 4g; Net Carbs: 2g; Protein: 3g MACROS – Fat: 50%; Protein: 17%; Carbs: 33%

STRAWBERRY WATERMELON GRANITAS

PREP TIME: 5 MINUTES, PLUS 6 TO 8 HOURS TO FREEZE

AIP-Reintroduction Phase: Keto Sweeteners (erythritol),
Low-Sugar Alcohol (vodka)

SERVES 6

Alcohol can be enjoyed in moderation on a keto diet, so treat yourself to a cold and refreshing granita. Each serving is packed with vitamin C and is the ultimate refresher to serve at summer parties! This drink takes 6 to 8 hours to freeze, so make sure to plan ahead and make it the night before.

1 cup chopped strawberries

½ cup chopped watermelon

1 cup vodka

½ cup filtered water

1 tablespoon lemon juice

¼ cup granular erythritol
(like Swerve brand)

1. In a blender, blend strawberries, watermelon, vodka, water, lemon juice, and erythritol together until the mixture is smooth.

2. Pour the mixture in a 9-by 13-inch baking dish and cover it with plastic wrap.

3. Freeze the mixture for 6 to 8 hours before serving or until frozen, then use a fork to scrape it into ice shavings.

4. Immediately scoop the ice shavings into glasses and serve.

Tip: Choose a vodka that is gluten-free, such as Tito's.

Per Serving Calories: 98; Total Fat: 0g; Total Carbs: 3g; Fiber: 1g; Net Carbs: 2g; Protein: 0g MACROS – Fat: 1%; Protein: 1%; Carbs: 11%; Alcohol: 87%

BLACKBERRY AND ROSEMARY EARL GREY VODKAS

PREP TIME: 10 MINUTES | COOK TIME: 5 MINUTES

AIP-Reintroduction Phase: Keto Sweeteners (erythritol),
Low-Sugar Alcohol (vodka)

SERVES 4

Fruity and herby, this pleasing adult beverage is wonderful any time of the year. Garnish each glass with blackberries and a sprig of rosemary when serving them at parties.

6 Earl Grey tea bags

4 cups filtered water

2 tablespoons granular erythritol (like Swerve brand)

½ cup blackberries

2 large rosemary sprigs

¼ cup ice, plus more for serving

¼ cup full-fat coconut milk

6 ounces vodka

1. In a medium saucepan, heat the tea bags, water, and erythritol over medium heat for 3 minutes.
2. Remove the tea bags.
3. While the tea is still hot, add the blackberries and rosemary to the saucepan.
4. Using the end of a wooden spoon, muddle the berries until they are completely mashed.
5. Strain the mixture into a pitcher and add ¼ cup ice to allow the mixture to cool.
6. Stir in the coconut milk and vodka.
7. Fill 4 glasses with ice, pour the drink into each glass, and serve.

Tips: Choose a vodka that is gluten-free, such as Tito's. Or omit the vodka altogether to make this a virgin mocktail.

Swaps: Feel free to substitute the coconut milk for heavy cream if you have successfully reintroduced dairy.

Per Serving Calories: 132; Total Fat: 3g; Total Carbs: 2g; Fiber: 1g; Net Carbs: 1g; Protein: 1g MACROS - Fat: 20%; Protein: 1%; Carbs: 6%; Alcohol: 73%

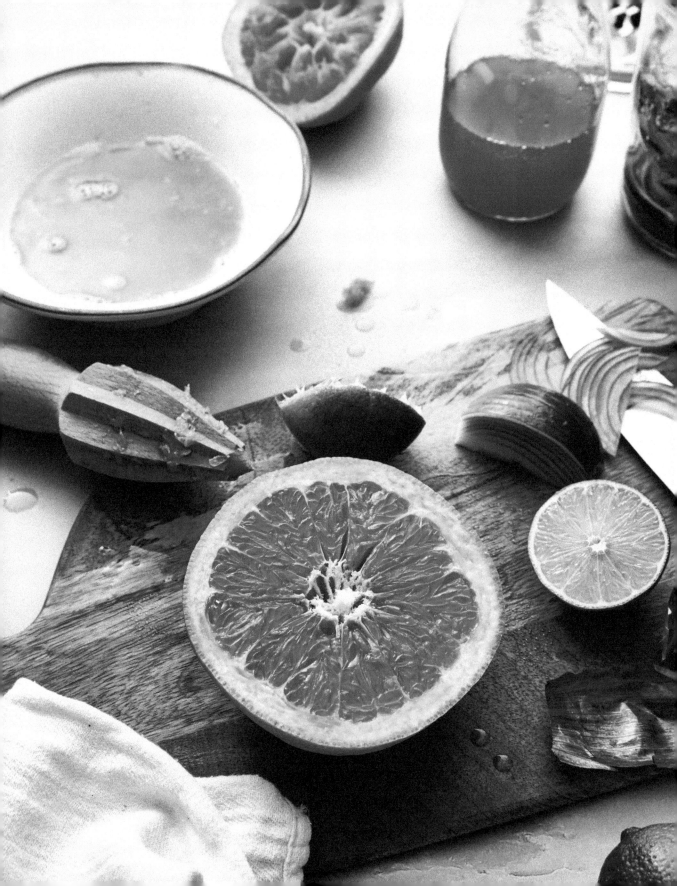

Chapter 11

STAPLES, SAUCES, AND DRESSINGS

BASIL PESTO

PREP TIME: 5 MINUTES

AIP-Elimination Phase Compliant

MAKES ¾ CUP

Basil Pesto is a versatile sauce that you can use to drizzle over seafood or vegetables. Traditional pesto is made with pine nuts and Parmesan. Our version replaces these ingredients with Kalamata olives to make this recipe AIP-Elimination Phase compliant. We like to make a big batch on the weekend to use throughout the week.

2 cups fresh basil

¼ cup Kalamata
  olives, pitted

4 cloves garlic

½ teaspoon salt

¼ cup extra-virgin olive oil

1. Put the basil, olives, garlic, and salt in a food processor or blender; process to combine.

2. Slowly pour in the olive oil and pulse until smooth.

Tip: Store in a sealed container in the refrigerator for up to 7 days.

Swap: Feel free to substitute the olives with 1 tablespoon pine nuts and 2 tablespoons Parmesan cheese if these have been successfully reintroduced.

Per Serving (1 tablespoon) Calories: 45; Total Fat: 5g; Total Carbs: 1g; Fiber: 0g; Net Carbs: 1g; Protein: 0g MACROS – Fat: 93%; Protein: 2%; Carbs: 5%

CHIMICHURRI SAUCE

PREP TIME: 5 MINUTES

AIP-Elimination Phase Compliant

MAKES 1 CUP

Chimichurri is a vibrant Argentinian sauce that packs a ton of flavor! This sauce pairs perfectly with steak, chicken, or seafood.

1 cup fresh parsley, chopped

½ cup fresh cilantro, chopped

4 cloves garlic, minced

1 teaspoon salt

1½ teaspoons dried oregano

¼ cup red wine vinegar

½ cup extra-virgin olive oil

1. Put the parsley, cilantro, garlic, salt, oregano, and vinegar in a food processor or blender; process to combine.

2. Slowly pour in the olive oil and pulse until smooth.

Tip: Store in a sealed container in the refrigerator for up to 7 days.

Swaps: Add ½ teaspoon cumin and ½ teaspoon crushed red pepper, if you have successfully reintroduced these spices.

Per Serving (2 tablespoons) Calories: 127; Total Fat: 14g; Total Carbs: 1g; Fiber: 0g; Net Carbs: 1g; Protein: 0g MACROS · Fat: 95%; Protein: 1%; Carbs: 4%

GREEK VINAIGRETTE

PREP TIME: 5 MINUTES

AIP-Elimination Phase Compliant

MAKES 1½ CUPS

The traditional flavors of Greece, including oregano, garlic, and red wine vinegar, come together in this vibrant salad dressing.

½ cup red wine vinegar

2 cloves garlic, minced

2 teaspoons dried oregano

1 teaspoon dried thyme

½ teaspoon salt

1 cup extra-virgin olive oil

1. In a small bowl, whisk the vinegar, oregano, garlic, thyme, and salt vigorously.

2. Slowly pour in the olive oil and continue to whisk until fully combined.

Tips: Store this salad dressing in a sealed container in the refrigerator for up to 7 days. Shake the container before using.

Per Serving (2 tablespoons) Calories: 161; Total Fat: 18g; Total Carbs: 0g; Fiber: 0g; Net Carbs: 0g; Protein: 0g MACROS - Fat: 99%; Protein: 0%; Carbs: 1%

AUTOIMMUNE KETO HOUSE DRESSING

PREP TIME: 5 MINUTES

AIP-Elimination Phase Compliant

MAKES 1 CUP

We call this the Autoimmune Keto House Dressing because we use this dressing ALL THE TIME. It will soon be your go-to salad dressing!

3 tablespoons
  balsamic vinegar

2 tablespoons apple
  cider vinegar

½ teaspoon garlic powder

½ teaspoon onion powder

½ teaspoon dried basil

½ teaspoon salt

1 teaspoon raw
  honey (optional)

⅔ cup extra-virgin olive oil

1. In a small bowl, whisk the vinegars, garlic powder, onion powder, basil, salt, and honey (if using) vigorously.

2. Slowly pour in the olive oil and continue to whisk until fully combined.

Tips: Store this salad dressing in a sealed container in the refrigerator for up to 7 days. Shake the container before using.

Swap: To lower the carb content, you can swap out the honey for 1 teaspoon of erythritol or 4 drops liquid stevia extract if these have been successfully reintroduced.

Per Serving (2 tablespoons) Calories: 164; Total Fat: 18g; Total Carbs: 1g; Fiber: 0g; Net Carbs: 1g; Protein: 0g MACROS · Fat: 99%; Protein: 0%; Carbs: 1%

COCONUT YOGURT

PREP TIME: 15 MINUTES | COOK TIME: 48 HOURS

AIP-Elimination Phase Compliant

MAKES 3 CUPS

Most store-bought coconut yogurts have added sugars or thickeners, so we like to make our own with just 4 ingredients, a mason jar, and an oven. The key to making yogurt is using probiotic capsules. Make sure the probiotics are gluten-free and contain one or more of the following bacteria strains: *Lactobacillus acidophilus*, *Bifidobacterium bifidum*, *Bifidobacterium lactis*, and *Streptococcus thermophilus*.

2 cups full-fat coconut milk

1 cup coconut cream

1 teaspoon beef gelatin (like Great Lakes or Vital Proteins brand)

2 probiotic capsules

1. Turn the oven light on to add a small amount of heat to your oven.

2. Fill a quart-sized mason jar with boiling filtered water and set aside.

3. In a saucepan, combine the coconut milk and coconut cream over medium heat until it reaches 110°F.

4. Sprinkle the gelatin into the coconut mixture and whisk vigorously until combined.

5. Remove the saucepan from heat.

6. Break the probiotic capsules open and add the capsule contents into the coconut mixture and whisk to combine.

7. Pour the water out of the mason jar and add the coconut mixture to the empty jar.

8. Screw the lid onto the jar and immediately place in the oven near the oven light.

9. Keep the jar in the oven for 24 hours, making sure the oven light remains on the entire time.

10. After 24 hours, transfer the mason jar to the refrigerator to thicken for an additional 24 hours.

11. After 24 hours in the refrigerator, feel free to enjoy!

Tips: Put a sticky note on the outside of your oven with a reminder to not open the oven or turn off the oven light. Store in the refrigerator for up to 7 days.

Per Serving (½ cup) Calories: 284; Total Fat: 30g; Total Carbs: 5g; Fiber: 1g; Net Carbs: 4g; Protein: 4g MACROS - Fat: 88%; Protein: 5%; Carbs: 7%

SWEET HORSERADISH CREAM

PREP TIME: 5 MINUTES

AIP-Elimination Phase Compliant

MAKES 1½ CUPS

One of the best ways to get a kick of heat into an AIP-compliant dish is with horseradish. Serve this Sweet Horseradish Cream with steak or our Garlic Rosemary Zucchini Chips (page 87). This sauce keeps for up to 5 days in an airtight container in the refrigerator.

½ cup fresh horseradish, peeled and grated

1 cup plain unsweetened Coconut Yogurt (page 178)

1 tablespoon apple cider vinegar

1½ teaspoons raw honey

¼ teaspoon salt

Mix together the horseradish, yogurt, vinegar, honey, and salt in a small bowl.

Tips: Use a knife to peel off the skin of the horseradish root and then use the medium grate option on your box grater to finely grate it. Keep your horseradish root refrigerated before grating to help to prevent it from stinging your eyes! If you don't have time to make the homemade Coconut Yogurt on page 178, feel free to use a store-bought version. Just make sure the only ingredients on the food label are coconut, water, and probiotic cultures. We like the brands Anita's and GT's CocoYo.

Swaps: You can substitute the coconut yogurt for an equal amount of sour cream if you have successfully reintroduced dairy. To lower the carb content, swap out the honey for 1 teaspoon of erythritol if it has been successfully reintroduced.

Per Serving (¼ cup) Calories: 144; Total Fat: 12g; Total Carbs: 8g; Fiber: 1g; Net Carbs: 7g; Protein: 1g MACROS · Fat: 75%; Protein: 3%; Carbs: 22%

CUCUMBER TZATZIKI

PREP TIME: 5 MINUTES

AIP-Elimination Phase Compliant

MAKES 1 CUP

Tzatziki is a creamy, cucumber-infused, tangy dip that is perfect with our Greek Meatball Lettuce Wraps (page 133) or as a dip for cucumbers, carrots, and celery.

¾ cup plain unsweetened Coconut Yogurt (page 178)

1 tablespoon extra-virgin olive oil

½ tablespoon fresh mint, chopped

½ tablespoon fresh dill, chopped

½ tablespoon lemon juice

1 clove garlic, minced

½ teaspoon salt

1 cup cucumber, grated and liquid squeezed out through paper towels

1. Mix the yogurt, olive oil, mint, dill, lemon juice, garlic, and salt in a small bowl.

2. Add in the grated cucumbers and stir until fully incorporated.

Tips: One large cucumber should yield 2 cups, so you only need to grate half the cucumber. Use a cheese grater to grate the cucumber, and there is no need to peel or seed the cucumber first. Store in a sealed container in the refrigerator for up to 5 days. If you don't have time to make the homemade Coconut Yogurt on page 178, feel free to use a store-bought version. Just make sure the only ingredients on the food label are coconut, water, and probiotic cultures. We like the brands Anita's and GT's CocoYo.

Per Serving (¼ cup) Calories: 167; Total Fat: 15g; Total Carbs: 6g; Fiber: 1g; Net Carbs: 5g; Protein: 2g MACROS · Fat: 81%; Protein: 5%; Carbs: 14%

GRAPEFRUIT RED ONIONS

PREP TIME: 5 MINUTES, 12 HOURS TO CHILL

AIP-Elimination Phase Compliant

2 CUPS

These Grapefruit Red Onions are our version of pickled onions. The citrus juices and red wine vinegar contribute incredible flavor. We love adding these to salads and taco bowls.

1 cup grapefruit juice,
   fresh squeezed

¼ cup lime juice,
   fresh squeezed

1 cup red wine vinegar

¼ teaspoon salt

¼ teaspoon garlic powder

1 medium red onion,
   thinly sliced

1. Combine the grapefruit juice, lime juice, and red wine vinegar in a large mason jar.

2. Add the salt and garlic powder to the jar and stir to combine.

3. Add the red onion slices to the jar, making sure all the onions are submerged into the liquid.

4. Put in the refrigerator to pickle for at least 12 hours before serving.

Tip: Store the onions in the refrigerator for up to 10 days.

Per Serving (¼ cup) Calories: 8; Total Fat: 0g; Total Carbs: 2g; Fiber: 0g; Net Carbs: 2g; Protein: 0g MACROS · Fat: 2%; Protein: 6%; Carbs: 92%

SEAFOOD SEASONING BLEND

PREP TIME: 5 MINUTES

AIP-Reintroduction Phase: Nightshades (paprika, cayenne pepper),
Non-AIP Spices (black pepper, mustard, allspice)

2 TABLESPOONS

Many store-bought seasoning blends have added fillers or sugar, so we like to make our own combinations. Here are a few of our favorites, but feel free to mix and match based on what spices you have successfully introduced.

1 tablespoon celery salt
2 teaspoons paprika
1 teaspoon ground mustard
¼ teaspoon black pepper
¼ teaspoon allspice
¼ teaspoon cayenne pepper
⅛ teaspoon ground
   cinnamon

1. In a small bowl, combine the celery salt, paprika, ground mustard, black pepper, allspice, cayenne pepper, and cinnamon.

2. Store in a sealed container at room temperature for up to 6 months.

Seafood Seasoning Per Serving (1 teaspoon) Calories: 4; Total Fat: 0g; Total Carbs: 1g; Fiber: 0g; Net Carbs: 1g; Protein: 0g MACROS - Fat: 0%; Protein: 0%; Carbs: 100%

CAJUN SEASONING BLEND

PREP TIME: 5 MINUTES

AIP-Reintroduction Phase: Nightshades (paprika, cayenne pepper),
Non-AIP Spices (black pepper, mustard, allspice)

2 TABLESPOONS

1 tablespoon paprika

½ tablespoon garlic powder

½ teaspoon onion powder

½ teaspoon salt

½ teaspoon black pepper

½ teaspoon cayenne pepper

1. In a small bowl, combine the paprika, garlic powder, onion powder, salt, black pepper, and cayenne pepper.

2. Store in a sealed container at room temperature for up to 6 months.

Cajun Seasoning Per Serving (1 teaspoon) Calories: 5; Total Fat: 0g; Total Carbs: 1g; Fiber: 0g; Net Carbs: 1g; Protein: 0g MACROS · Fat: 0%; Protein: 1%; Carbs: 99%

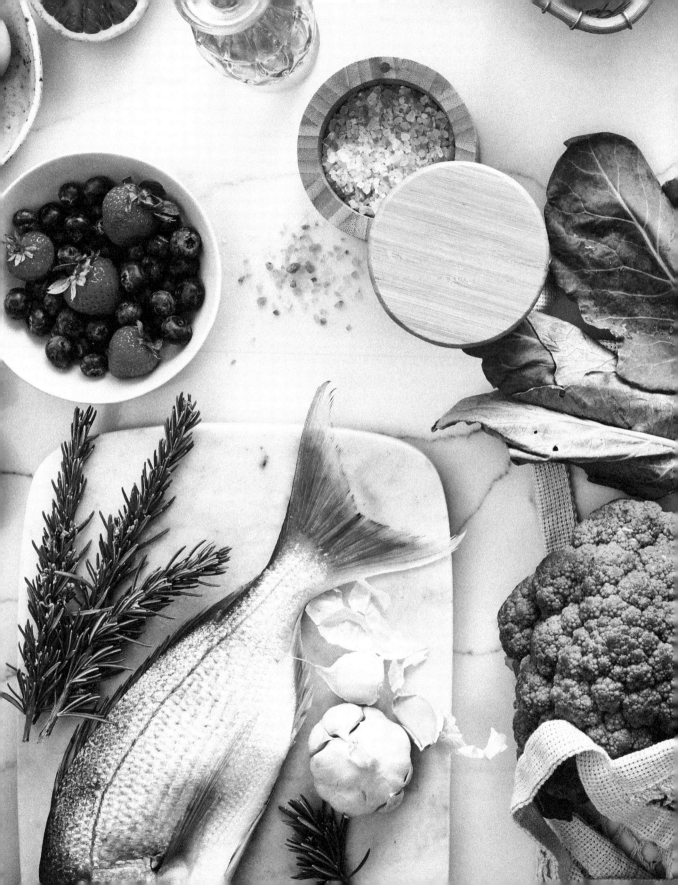

MEASUREMENT CONVERSIONS

VOLUME EQUIVALENTS (LIQUID)		
US STANDARD	US STANDARD (OUNCES)	METRIC
2 TABLE SPOONS	1 FL. OZ.	30 ML
¼ CUP	2 FL. OZ.	60 ML
½ CUP	4 FL. OZ	120 ML
1 CUP	8 FL. OZ.	240 ML
1½ CUPS	12 FL. OZ.	355 ML
2 CUPS OR 1 PINT	16 FL. OZ.	475 ML
4 CUPS OR 1 QUART	32 FL. OZ.	1 L

VOLUME EQUIVALENTS (DRY)	
US STANDARD	METRIC (APPROXIMATE)
⅛ TEASPOON	0.5 ML
¼ TEASPOON	2 ML
½ TEASPOON	4 ML
¾ TEASPOON	5 ML
1 TEASPOON	15 ML
¼ CUP	59 ML
⅓ CUP	79 ML
½ CUP	118 ML
⅔ CUP	156 ML
¾ CUP	177 ML
1 CUP	235 ML
2 CUPS OR 1 PINT	475 ML
3 CUPS	700 ML
4CUPS OR 1 QUART	1 L

WEIGHT EQUIVALENTS	
US STANDARD	METRIC (APPROXIMATE)
½ OUNCE	15 G
1 OUNCE	30 G
2 OUNCES	60 G
4 OUNCES	115 G
0 OUNCES	225 G
12 OUNCES	340 G
16 OUNCES OR 1 POUND	455 G
OVEN TEMPRATURES	
FAHRENHEIT (F)	CELSIUS (C) (APPROXIMATE)
250°F	120°C
300°F	150°C
325°F	165°C
350°F	180°C
375°F	190°C
400°F	200°C
425°F	220°C
450°F	230°C

RESOURCES

Looking for more Autoimmune Keto information?

CleanKetoLifestyle.com: Head over to our website for more recipes and resources. We also offer group programs and one-on-one coaching to assist people in implementing Autoimmune Keto.

Clean Keto Lifestyle: The Complete Guide to Transforming Your Life and Health by Karissa Long: This is the first book written by Karissa and it is a perfect companion to Autoimmune Keto. The book includes 75+ keto recipes, 5 weeks of meal plans, exercise routines, and specific advice on how to eat a ketogenic diet when you are out in social situations.

The Paleo Approach: Reverse Autoimmune Disease and Heal Your Body by Sarah D. Ballantyne, Ph.D.: Ballantyne breaks down the science and medical research on why you should follow the autoimmune protocol if you have an autoimmune disease.

The Big Book of Ketogenic Diet Cooking by Jen Fisch: This cookbook is filled with 200 keto-friendly recipes to add to your rotation and ensure you have plenty of variety in your diet.

The Easy 5-Ingredient Ketogenic Diet Cookbook by Jen Fisch: Simplify your life with a cookbook that will have you eating tasty keto dishes—using just five ingredients or less!

RECIPE INDEX

INDEX

ACKNOWLEDGMENTS

First and foremost, thank you to our amazing Clean Keto Lifestyle community, which inspires us every single day with incredible healing stories and transformations. You are the reason we wrote this book. Your success motivated us to share our Autoimmune Keto approach with as many people as possible.

To our families who have given us so much support throughout our journeys with our respective autoimmune diseases. From taking us to endless doctor's appointments, caring for us as we struggled with the debilitating symptoms, and being there every step of the way as we embarked on implementing Autoimmune Keto. You were there with us for the good and the bad and we will forever be grateful for your unwavering love.

ABOUT THE AUTHORS

About Karissa

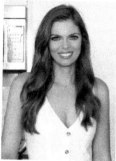

As a global health coach and ketogenic expert for women, Karissa has been living the keto life and helping others live it for almost a decade with her proprietary keto-coaching programs, courses, and meal plans. Karissa found the ketogenic diet during her struggle with ulcerative colitis, and has taken everything she learned through her own health journey and made it her mission to help others achieve optimal health.

Karissa is also the best-selling author of *Clean Keto Lifestyle*. What makes her method different from all the other keto programs out there is that she is all about putting health first and foremost. She focuses on doing the ketogenic diet the right way with a menu full of fresh, clean, nutrient-dense fats, proteins, and vegetables, free of processed foods and artificial ingredients.

About Katie

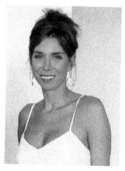

Katie is an executive chef and recipe developer extraordinaire who has taken her incredible skills in the kitchen and parlayed them into her passion for living a keto lifestyle. Katie discovered the ketogenic diet when she was suffering from multiple autoimmune diseases, including Hashimoto's Thyroiditis, Postural Orthostatic Tachycardia Syndrome, and Ankylosing Spondylitis. Her worst symptoms were fatigue, heart palpitations, and arthritis.

After years of trying different treatment methods in an attempt to control her autoimmune diseases, the Autoimmune Keto approach was the *first* thing that actually worked! She found that ridding her body of sugars and embracing nutritious fats and vegetables were the key to her success. Amazed by her health transformation, Katie set out to make cooking keto easy, attainable, and BEAUTIFUL!

f P O Follow us on Facebook, Pinterest, and Instagram @cleanketolifestyle

www.cleanketolifestyle.com

CPSIA information can be obtained
at www.ICGtesting.com
Printed in the USA
LVHW070048031219
639020LV00002B/1/P

9 781646 110384